Super Easy
DSM5-TR

The fundamental guide for students and
professionals in mental health

© Copyright 2024 - All rights reserved.

Table of Contents

Introduction

Welcome to *Super Easy DSM-5-TR*, your essential guide for mastering the DSM-5-TR (Diagnostic and Statistical Manual of Mental Disorders, Fifth Edition, Text Revision). This book has been meticulously designed to simplify the complexities of mental health diagnostics, making it an invaluable resource for students, clinicians, and mental health professionals. Our aim is to streamline your understanding and application of DSM-5-TR criteria, providing practical tools and clear explanations to enhance your diagnostic skills.

Purpose of the Book

The DSM-5-TR is a comprehensive manual used for diagnosing mental health disorders, but its breadth can often be overwhelming. *Super Easy DSM-5-TR* seeks to demystify this extensive manual by breaking down its content into clear, manageable sections. This guide is designed to:

1. **Clarify Complex Information**: By distilling detailed diagnostic criteria into understandable terms, we simplify the process of mastering DSM-5-TR concepts.
2. **Enhance Learning and Recall**: Utilizing mnemonics, cheat sheets, and practical examples, we aim to boost your ability to remember and effectively apply diagnostic criteria.

3. **Support Practical Application**: Through diagnostic flowcharts and case studies, we provide practical tools that facilitate real-world diagnosis and clinical decision-making.

How to Use This Book

Super Easy DSM-5-TR is organized to guide you systematically through the diagnostic process:

1. **Part I: Understanding DSM-5-TR** – This introductory section covers the DSM-5-TR's history, purpose, and structure. It also highlights key changes introduced in the latest edition, providing a solid foundation for the content that follows.
2. **Part II: Core Disorders (Condensed)** – This section delves into major categories of mental health disorders, including neurodevelopmental, mood, and anxiety disorders, among others. Each disorder is presented with:
   - **Key Features**: Essential characteristics that define each disorder.
   - **Simplified Diagnostic Criteria**: Streamlined criteria for easier application.
   - **Case Studies**: Practical examples illustrating the application of criteria in clinical settings.
3. **Part III: Study Aids and Practice** – Designed to reinforce your understanding and application of DSM-5-TR criteria, this section includes:
   - **Cheat Sheets**: Detailed mnemonics and simplified diagnostic criteria for quick reference.

- o **Practice Exams**: Sample questions to test your knowledge and comprehension.
- o **Diagnostic Flowcharts**: Visual aids to help organize and simplify the diagnostic process.
4. **Part IV: Online and Interactive Resources** – Enhance your learning with additional online tools:
   - o **Quizzes**: Interactive quizzes to assess your knowledge and track progress.
   - o **Flashcards**: Printable and digital flashcards for rapid review.
   - o **Audio Summaries**: Concise audio summaries of key concepts to support auditory learning.

Overview of Bonuses and Online Resources

In addition to the book, you will have access to a variety of online resources designed to complement your learning:

1. **Interactive Quizzes**: Available on the book's website, these quizzes offer a dynamic way to test your understanding of DSM-5-TR criteria, providing immediate feedback to help you gauge your grasp of the material.
2. **Flashcards**: Both printable and digital formats are provided for quick review and reinforcement of key diagnostic criteria and concepts.
3. **Audio Summaries**: For auditory learners, concise audio summaries of essential topics are available, allowing for convenient review and reinforcement of key concepts.

Enjoy the Journey

Embarking on the journey to mastering DSM-5-TR is both a challenge and an opportunity for professional growth. As you delve into the complexities of mental health diagnostics, remember that every step you take brings you closer to a deeper understanding and more effective practice.

This guide is designed to support you every step of the way, offering clear explanations, practical tools, and interactive resources to enhance your learning experience. Approach each section with curiosity and openness, and take the time to engage with the material fully. The path to mastering DSM-5-TR is an ongoing process, and each chapter you complete adds to your expertise and confidence.

We encourage you to explore the book thoroughly, make use of the supplementary online resources, and apply the knowledge in practical settings. As you advance through *Super Easy DSM-5-TR*, we hope you find both the process and the outcomes rewarding. Embrace the journey with a sense of discovery and professionalism, and let this guide be a valuable companion in your pursuit of excellence in mental health diagnostics.

Welcome to a more accessible and effective way to understand and apply DSM-5-TR criteria. Enjoy the journey and the professional growth it brings!

PART I:

Understanding DSM-5-TR

Introduction to DSM-5-TR

The Diagnostic and Statistical Manual of Mental Disorders, Fifth Edition, Text Revision (DSM-5-TR) is a comprehensive classification system for mental disorders. It is used by clinicians, researchers, and policymakers to diagnose and classify mental health conditions. The DSM-5-TR provides standardized criteria for the diagnosis of mental disorders, ensuring consistency and reliability in the assessment and treatment of patients. This section will introduce you to the DSM-5-TR, its history, purpose, and significance in the field of mental health.

The DSM-5-TR is an essential tool for mental health professionals. It aids in the accurate diagnosis of mental health conditions, facilitating effective treatment and management. The manual's standardized criteria help reduce variability in diagnosis, ensuring that patients receive consistent and evidence-based care. Additionally, the DSM-5-TR plays a crucial role in research, providing a common framework for studying mental disorders and their treatment.

The DSM-5-TR is also important for policymakers and insurance companies. By providing clear and standardized diagnostic criteria, the manual helps define mental health conditions for legal and insurance purposes. This ensures that patients receive the necessary coverage and support for their mental health needs.

Understanding the DSM-5-TR is vital for anyone involved in the field of mental health. Whether you are a clinician, researcher, or student, a thorough knowledge of the DSM-5-TR will enhance your ability to diagnose and treat mental health conditions effectively. This section provides an overview of the DSM-5-TR, helping you navigate its structure and understand its key components.

History and Purpose

The DSM has a long history dating back to the 1950s when the first edition was published by the American Psychiatric Association (APA). The purpose of the DSM is to provide a common language and standard criteria for the classification of mental disorders. Over the decades, the DSM has undergone several revisions to reflect advances in research and changes in clinical practice.

The first edition of the DSM, published in 1952, was a modest document with a limited number of mental disorders. It was based on the best available knowledge at the time but lacked the scientific rigor of later editions. As the field of psychiatry evolved, so did the DSM. The second edition, published in 1968, included more disorders and provided more detailed descriptions.

The third edition, published in 1980, marked a significant shift in the DSM's approach. It introduced a multi-axial system for diagnosing mental disorders, considering various aspects of a patient's condition. This edition was also more research-based, reflecting the growing emphasis on evidence-based practice in psychiatry.

The fourth edition, published in 1994, built on the foundation of the third edition. It included more disorders, updated diagnostic criteria, and improved organization. The DSM-IV-TR, a text revision published in 2000, made further refinements based on new research and clinical experience.

The DSM-5, published in 2013, represented another major update. It eliminated the multi-axial system, integrated new research findings, and introduced several new disorders. The DSM-5-TR, the latest text revision, builds on the DSM-5, incorporating the latest research and clinical insights to provide the most up-to-date and comprehensive classification of mental disorders.

Structure and Components

The DSM-5-TR is organized into three main sections. The first section provides an introduction to the manual, including instructions on how to use it. This section outlines the rationale behind the DSM-5-TR's organization and provides guidance on diagnosing mental disorders.

The second section contains the diagnostic criteria and codes for all recognized mental disorders. These criteria are organized into categories based on similarities in symptoms and underlying features. Each disorder is described in detail, including diagnostic criteria, associated features, prevalence, development and course, risk and prognostic factors, and diagnostic markers.

The third section includes tools and techniques to enhance the use of the manual. This section contains assessment measures, cultural formulations, and alternative diagnostic models. It provides guidance on using these tools to improve the accuracy and reliability of diagnoses.

The DSM-5-TR also includes several appendices. These appendices provide additional information on various topics, such as the classification of mental disorders, glossary of technical terms, and updates on future research directions. The appendices are valuable resources for clinicians and researchers seeking a deeper understanding of the DSM-5-TR.

Key Changes in DSM-5-TR

The DSM-5-TR introduces several key changes and updates to the DSM-5. These changes reflect the latest research findings and clinical insights, ensuring that the manual remains current and relevant. Some of the most significant changes include updates to diagnostic criteria, the introduction of new disorders, and the reclassification of existing disorders.

One of the key updates in the DSM-5-TR is the refinement of diagnostic criteria for several disorders. These updates are based on new research and aim to improve the accuracy and reliability of diagnoses. For example, the criteria for autism spectrum disorder have been updated to reflect the latest understanding of the condition's symptoms and developmental trajectory.

The DSM-5-TR also introduces new disorders that were not included in the DSM-5. These new disorders reflect emerging research and clinical practice, addressing conditions that were previously unrecognized or poorly understood. For example, the DSM-5-TR includes a new category for internet gaming disorder, recognizing the growing impact of digital addiction on mental health.

In addition to introducing new disorders, the DSM-5-TR reclassifies several existing disorders to better reflect current knowledge. For example, some disorders have been moved to different categories based on new evidence about their underlying features and relationships to other conditions. These reclassifications aim to improve the manual's organization and enhance the clinician's ability to diagnose and treat mental disorders effectively.

The DSM-5-TR also includes updates to the cultural formulation section, providing more detailed guidance on assessing and diagnosing mental disorders across diverse cultural contexts. This update reflects the growing recognition of the importance of cultural competence in mental health practice and aims to improve the accuracy and relevance of diagnoses for individuals from diverse backgrounds.

Overall, the DSM-5-TR represents a significant advancement in the classification and diagnosis of mental disorders. By incorporating the latest research and clinical insights, the manual provides a comprehensive and up-to-date resource for mental health professionals. Understanding these key changes and updates is essential for anyone using the DSM-5-TR in clinical practice or research.

PART II:

Core Disorders (Condensed)

Neurodevelopmental Disorders

Key Features

Neurodevelopmental disorders are a group of conditions with onset in the developmental period. These disorders typically manifest early in development, often before the child enters grade school, and are characterized by developmental deficits that produce impairments of personal, social, academic, or occupational functioning. The range of developmental deficits varies from very specific limitations of learning or control of executive functions to global impairments of social skills or intelligence.

Simplified Diagnostic Criteria

1. Autism Spectrum Disorder (ASD)

- **Persistent deficits in social communication and social interaction:**
    - Deficits in social-emotional reciprocity (e.g., abnormal social approach, failure to initiate or respond to social interactions).
    - Deficits in nonverbal communicative behaviors (e.g., poorly integrated verbal and nonverbal communication, abnormalities in eye contact and body language).
    - Deficits in developing, maintaining, and understanding relationships (e.g., difficulties adjusting behavior to suit various social contexts, difficulty sharing imaginative play).

22

- **Restricted, repetitive patterns of behavior, interests, or activities** (at least two of the following):
  - Stereotyped or repetitive motor movements, use of objects, or speech (e.g., simple motor stereotypies, lining up toys or flipping objects).
  - Insistence on sameness, inflexible adherence to routines, or ritualized patterns of verbal or nonverbal behavior (e.g., extreme distress at small changes, difficulties with transitions).
  - Highly restricted, fixated interests that are abnormal in intensity or focus (e.g., strong attachment to or preoccupation with unusual objects).
  - Hyper- or hyporeactivity to sensory input or unusual interest in sensory aspects of the environment (e.g., apparent indifference to pain/temperature, adverse response to specific sounds or textures).
- **Symptoms must be present in the early developmental period** (but may not become fully manifest until social demands exceed limited capacities or may be masked by learned strategies later in life).
- **Symptoms cause clinically significant impairment** in social, occupational, or other important areas of current functioning.
- **These disturbances are not better explained by** intellectual disability or global developmental delay. Intellectual disability and autism spectrum disorder frequently co-occur; to make comorbid diagnoses of autism spectrum disorder and intellectual disability, social

communication should be below that expected for general developmental level.

Case Study

Case Study: James

James is a 5-year-old boy who has recently been diagnosed with Autism Spectrum Disorder (ASD). His parents noticed that James was not meeting his developmental milestones, particularly in the areas of communication and social interaction. He rarely made eye contact, did not respond to his name, and had difficulty engaging in play with other children. Instead, he preferred to play alone, often lining up his toy cars in a precise order and becoming very upset if they were moved.

James exhibited repetitive behaviors, such as hand flapping and spinning objects. He also showed a strong preference for routine and became distressed with any changes to his daily schedule. His speech was limited, and he often echoed phrases he heard others say (echolalia) rather than using language to communicate his needs.

A comprehensive evaluation by a multidisciplinary team, including a psychologist, speech therapist, and occupational therapist, confirmed the diagnosis of ASD.

The evaluation included observations of James in various settings, parent interviews, and standardized assessment tools. The team recommended an individualized education program (IEP) to address James' specific needs, focusing on improving his communication skills, social interactions, and adaptive behaviors.

Through early intervention services, including speech therapy and applied behavior analysis (ABA), James has made significant progress.

He has started to use simple words to request items and engage in more interactive play with his peers. His parents have also learned strategies to support his development at home, such as using visual schedules and reinforcing positive behaviors.

Schizophrenia Spectrum and Other Psychotic Disorders

Key Features

Schizophrenia spectrum and other psychotic disorders are characterized by abnormalities in one or more of the following five domains: delusions, hallucinations, disorganized thinking (speech), grossly disorganized or abnormal motor behavior (including catatonia), and negative symptoms.

These disorders include schizophrenia, schizotypal (personality) disorder, brief psychotic disorder, schizophreniform disorder, schizoaffective disorder, and substance/medication-induced psychotic disorder.

Simplified Diagnostic Criteria

1. Schizophrenia

- **Two or more of the following symptoms**, each present for a significant portion of time during a 1-month period (or less if successfully treated). At least one of these should be (1), (2), or (3):
    1. Delusions (fixed false beliefs that are not amenable to change in light of conflicting evidence)
    2. Hallucinations (perception-like experiences that occur without an external stimulus, most commonly auditory)
    3. Disorganized speech (e.g., frequent derailment or incoherence)
    4. Grossly disorganized or catatonic behavior
    5. Negative symptoms (e.g., diminished emotional expression or avolition)
- **For a significant portion of the time since the onset of the disturbance**, the level of functioning in one or more major areas, such as work, interpersonal relations, or self-care, is markedly below the level achieved prior to the onset.
- **Continuous signs of the disturbance persist for at least 6 months.** This 6-month period must include at least 1 month of symptoms (or less if successfully treated) that meet Criterion A (i.e., active-phase symptoms) and may include periods of prodromal or residual symptoms. During these prodromal or residual periods, the signs of

the disturbance may be manifested by only negative symptoms or by two or more symptoms listed in Criterion A present in an attenuated form (e.g., odd beliefs, unusual perceptual experiences).

- **Schizoaffective disorder and depressive or bipolar disorder with psychotic features have been ruled out** because either (1) no major depressive or manic episodes have occurred concurrently with the active-phase symptoms, or (2) if mood episodes have occurred during active-phase symptoms, they have been present for a minority of the total duration of the active and residual periods of the illness.

- **The disturbance is not attributable to the physiological effects of a substance** (e.g., a drug of abuse, a medication) or another medical condition.

- **If there is a history of autism spectrum disorder or a communication disorder of childhood onset,** the additional diagnosis of schizophrenia is made only if prominent delusions or hallucinations, in addition to the other required symptoms of schizophrenia, are also present for at least 1 month (or less if successfully treated).

Case Study

Case Study: Maria

Maria is a 25-year-old woman who has been experiencing severe and disabling symptoms for the past year. Her family noticed changes in her behavior when she began to isolate herself, avoid social interactions, and express strange beliefs that others found perplexing. Maria claimed that she was being watched by secret government agents and that she could hear their voices discussing her every move.

Her symptoms included:

- **Delusions:** Maria was convinced that the government was monitoring her through hidden cameras in her home and that her neighbors were spying on her.
- **Hallucinations:** She reported hearing voices that were critical and derogatory, telling her she was worthless and should harm herself.
- **Disorganized Speech:** Conversations with Maria were often difficult to follow. She would jump from one topic to another without logical connections and sometimes speak in a jumbled or incoherent manner.
- **Grossly Disorganized Behavior:** Maria exhibited odd behaviors such as wearing multiple layers of clothing on a hot day and staring at a wall for hours.
- **Negative Symptoms:** She showed a lack of emotional expression, reduced motivation to perform daily activities, and neglected personal hygiene.

Maria's ability to function at work and maintain relationships deteriorated significantly. She was unable to hold a job, and her relationships with family and friends suffered due to her erratic behavior and intense paranoia.

After a comprehensive evaluation by a psychiatrist, Maria was diagnosed with schizophrenia. The diagnosis was based on the presence of multiple symptoms including delusions, hallucinations, disorganized speech, disorganized behavior, and negative symptoms persisting for more than six months.

Maria was started on antipsychotic medication, and her treatment plan included cognitive-behavioral therapy (CBT) to help her manage her symptoms and improve her functioning.

With ongoing treatment, Maria showed gradual improvement. Her delusions and hallucinations decreased in intensity, and she began to re-engage with her family and participate in social activities. Although she still faces challenges, Maria's condition has stabilized, and she continues to work with her treatment team to maintain her progress.

Bipolar and Related Disorders

Key Features

Bipolar and related disorders are characterized by mood swings that include emotional highs (mania or hypomania) and lows (depression).

These mood episodes are distinct periods of time with specific criteria that differentiate them from the individual's usual behavior.

The primary disorders in this category include Bipolar I Disorder, Bipolar II Disorder, Cyclothymic Disorder, and substance/medication-induced bipolar and related disorders.

Simplified Diagnostic Criteria

1. Bipolar I Disorder

- **Manic Episode** (required for diagnosis):
  - ○ A distinct period of abnormally and persistently elevated, expansive, or irritable mood and abnormally and persistently increased activity or energy, lasting at least 1 week and present most of the day, nearly every day (or any duration if hospitalization is necessary).
  - ○ During the period of mood disturbance and increased energy or activity, three (or more) of the following symptoms (four if the mood is only irritable) are present to a significant degree and represent a noticeable change from usual behavior:
    1. Inflated self-esteem or grandiosity
    2. Decreased need for sleep (e.g., feels rested after only 3 hours of sleep)
    3. More talkative than usual or pressure to keep talking
    4. Flight of ideas or subjective experience that thoughts are racing
    5. Distractibility (i.e., attention too easily drawn to unimportant or irrelevant external stimuli)
    6. Increase in goal-directed activity (either socially, at work or school, or sexually) or

psychomotor agitation (i.e., purposeless non-goal-directed activity)

7. Excessive involvement in activities that have a high potential for painful consequences (e.g., engaging in unrestrained buying sprees, sexual indiscretions, or foolish business investments)

o The mood disturbance is sufficiently severe to cause marked impairment in social or occupational functioning or to necessitate hospitalization to prevent harm to self or others, or there are psychotic features.

o The episode is not attributable to the physiological effects of a substance (e.g., a drug of abuse, a medication, other treatment) or another medical condition.

- **Hypomanic Episode** (not required for diagnosis, but often present):

  o A distinct period of abnormally and persistently elevated, expansive, or irritable mood and abnormally and persistently increased activity or energy, lasting at least 4 consecutive days and present most of the day, nearly every day.

  o During the period of mood disturbance and increased energy or activity, three (or more) of the following symptoms (four if the mood is only irritable) are present to a significant degree and represent a noticeable change from usual behavior:

31

1. Inflated self-esteem or grandiosity
2. Decreased need for sleep (e.g., feels rested after only 3 hours of sleep)
3. More talkative than usual or pressure to keep talking
4. Flight of ideas or subjective experience that thoughts are racing
5. Distractibility (i.e., attention too easily drawn to unimportant or irrelevant external stimuli)
6. Increase in goal-directed activity (either socially, at work or school, or sexually) or psychomotor agitation (i.e., purposeless non-goal-directed activity)
7. Excessive involvement in activities that have a high potential for painful consequences (e.g., engaging in unrestrained buying sprees, sexual indiscretions, or foolish business investments)

o The episode is associated with an unequivocal change in functioning that is uncharacteristic of the individual when not symptomatic.

o The disturbance in mood and the change in functioning are observable by others.

o The episode is not severe enough to cause marked impairment in social or occupational functioning or to necessitate hospitalization. If there are psychotic features, the episode is, by definition, manic.

- o The episode is not attributable to the physiological effects of a substance.
- **Major Depressive Episode** (not required for diagnosis, but often present):
  - o Five (or more) of the following symptoms have been present during the same 2-week period and represent a change from previous functioning; at least one of the symptoms is either (1) depressed mood or (2) loss of interest or pleasure.
    1. Depressed mood most of the day, nearly every day, as indicated by either subjective report (e.g., feels sad, empty, hopeless) or observation made by others (e.g., appears tearful).
    2. Markedly diminished interest or pleasure in all, or almost all, activities most of the day, nearly every day.
    3. Significant weight loss when not dieting or weight gain (e.g., a change of more than 5% of body weight in a month), or decrease or increase in appetite nearly every day.
    4. Insomnia or hypersomnia nearly every day.
    5. Psychomotor agitation or retardation nearly every day (observable by others, not merely subjective feelings of restlessness or being slowed down).
    6. Fatigue or loss of energy nearly every day.
    7. Feelings of worthlessness or excessive or inappropriate guilt (which may be

delusional) nearly every day (not merely self-reproach or guilt about being sick).

8. Diminished ability to think or concentrate, or indecisiveness, nearly every day (either by subjective account or as observed by others).

9. Recurrent thoughts of death (not just fear of dying), recurrent suicidal ideation without a specific plan, or a suicide attempt or a specific plan for committing suicide.

o   The symptoms cause clinically significant distress or impairment in social, occupational, or other important areas of functioning.

o   The episode is not attributable to the physiological effects of a substance or another medical condition.

Case Study

Case Study: John

John is a 30-year-old man who has experienced dramatic mood swings since his early twenties. His episodes are unpredictable, with periods of extreme happiness and energy followed by deep depression. During his manic episodes, John feels invincible. He has boundless energy, sleeps only a few hours each night, and engages in risky behaviors such as excessive spending and impulsive travel. His speech becomes rapid and difficult to interrupt, and his thoughts race from one idea to another.

During one manic episode, John quit his stable job, convinced that he could become a millionaire by starting his own business. He spent all his savings on this venture, only to abandon it weeks later when his mood shifted. His grandiose ideas and lack of planning led to financial ruin, and his relationships suffered due to his erratic behavior.

When his mood shifts to depression, John becomes lethargic and hopeless. He loses interest in activities he once enjoyed and isolates himself from friends and family. He struggles to get out of bed, experiences significant weight gain, and has recurrent thoughts of suicide. These depressive episodes can last for weeks or even months, severely impacting his ability to function in daily life. John's family urged him to seek help, and he was eventually diagnosed with Bipolar I Disorder. His psychiatrist prescribed mood stabilizers and antipsychotic medication to help manage his symptoms. John also began cognitive-behavioral therapy (CBT) to develop coping strategies and recognize early signs of mood changes.

With treatment, John has gained better control over his mood swings. He has learned to identify triggers and warning signs of both manic and depressive episodes. While he still experiences mood fluctuations, they are less severe, and he is better equipped to manage them. John's relationships and financial situation have also improved, allowing him to lead a more stable and fulfilling life.

Depressive Disorders

Key Features

Depressive disorders are characterized by persistent feelings of sadness, emptiness, or irritability, accompanied by somatic and cognitive changes that significantly impact an individual's ability to function. These disorders include Major Depressive Disorder (MDD), Persistent Depressive Disorder (Dysthymia), Disruptive Mood Dysregulation Disorder, and Premenstrual Dysphoric Disorder, among others.

Simplified Diagnostic Criteria

1. Major Depressive Disorder (MDD)

- **Five (or more) of the following symptoms** have been present during the same 2-week period and represent a change from previous functioning; at least one of the symptoms is either (1) depressed mood or (2) loss of interest or pleasure:
  1. Depressed mood most of the day, nearly every day, as indicated by either subjective report (e.g., feels sad, empty, hopeless) or observation made by others (e.g., appears tearful).
  2. Markedly diminished interest or pleasure in all, or almost all, activities most of the day, nearly every day.

3. Significant weight loss when not dieting or weight gain (e.g., a change of more than 5% of body weight in a month), or decrease or increase in appetite nearly every day.
4. Insomnia or hypersomnia nearly every day.
5. Psychomotor agitation or retardation nearly every day (observable by others, not merely subjective feelings of restlessness or being slowed down).
6. Fatigue or loss of energy nearly every day.
7. Feelings of worthlessness or excessive or inappropriate guilt (which may be delusional) nearly every day (not merely self-reproach or guilt about being sick).
8. Diminished ability to think or concentrate, or indecisiveness, nearly every day (either by subjective account or as observed by others).
9. Recurrent thoughts of death (not just fear of dying), recurrent suicidal ideation without a specific plan, or a suicide attempt or a specific plan for committing suicide.

- **The symptoms cause clinically significant distress or impairment** in social, occupational, or other important areas of functioning.
- **The episode is not attributable to the physiological effects of a substance** or another medical condition.
- **The occurrence of the major depressive episode is not better explained by schizoaffective disorder,** schizophrenia, schizophreniform disorder, delusional disorder, or other specified and unspecified schizophrenia spectrum and other psychotic disorders.

- **There has never been a manic episode or a hypomanic episode.**

Case Study

Case Study: Emily

Emily is a 28-year-old woman who has been experiencing persistent sadness and a loss of interest in activities she once enjoyed for the past several months. She reports feeling constantly tired, despite getting adequate sleep, and struggles to concentrate at work. Emily's appetite has decreased significantly, leading to a noticeable weight loss. She often feels worthless and guilty, blaming herself for things that are beyond her control.

Emily's symptoms include:

- **Depressed Mood:** Emily feels overwhelmingly sad and hopeless nearly every day. She finds it difficult to feel joy or pleasure in any aspect of her life.
- **Loss of Interest:** Activities that once brought her happiness, such as reading and spending time with friends, no longer interest her. She avoids social interactions and prefers to stay isolated.
- **Fatigue:** Despite sleeping for long hours, Emily feels exhausted and lacks the energy to perform daily tasks. Simple activities like getting out of bed and taking a shower feel like monumental efforts.

- **Weight Loss:** Emily has lost a significant amount of weight over the past few months due to a decreased appetite. She often skips meals because she has no desire to eat.
- **Feelings of Worthlessness:** Emily experiences intense feelings of guilt and worthlessness. She constantly criticizes herself and feels that she is a burden to others.
- **Difficulty Concentrating:** Emily struggles to focus on her work tasks and often makes mistakes. Her mind feels foggy, and she has difficulty making decisions.

Emily's symptoms have significantly impacted her ability to function at work and maintain relationships. She has missed several days of work and has withdrawn from her friends and family. Concerned about her well-being, Emily's sister encouraged her to seek help from a mental health professional.

After a thorough evaluation, Emily was diagnosed with Major Depressive Disorder. Her psychiatrist developed a treatment plan that included a combination of antidepressant medication and cognitive-behavioral therapy (CBT). The medication helped stabilize her mood, while CBT provided her with strategies to challenge negative thoughts and improve her coping skills.

Over time, Emily began to notice improvements in her mood and energy levels. She started to re-engage in activities she once enjoyed and gradually rebuilt her social connections. Although recovery was not immediate, Emily's commitment to her treatment plan and support from her therapist and family played a crucial role in her progress.

Emily's case highlights the importance of recognizing the signs of depression and seeking professional help. With appropriate treatment and support, individuals with Major Depressive Disorder can experience significant improvements in their quality of life and overall functioning.

Anxiety Disorders

Key Features

Anxiety disorders are characterized by excessive fear and anxiety and related behavioral disturbances. Fear is the emotional response to real or perceived imminent threat, whereas anxiety is anticipation of future threat. Anxiety disorders can lead to significant impairment in social, occupational, and other important areas of functioning. This category includes disorders such as Generalized Anxiety Disorder (GAD), Panic Disorder, Social Anxiety Disorder, Specific Phobias, and Agoraphobia.

Simplified Diagnostic Criteria

1. Generalized Anxiety Disorder (GAD)

- **Excessive anxiety and worry (apprehensive expectation)** occurring more days than not for at least 6 months, about a number of events or activities (such as work or school performance).

- The individual finds it difficult to control the worry.
- The anxiety and worry are associated with three (or more) of the following six symptoms (with at least some symptoms having been present for more days than not for the past 6 months):
    1. Restlessness or feeling keyed up or on edge
    2. Being easily fatigued
    3. Difficulty concentrating or mind going blank
    4. Irritability
    5. Muscle tension
    6. Sleep disturbance (difficulty falling or staying asleep, or restless, unsatisfying sleep)
- The anxiety, worry, or physical symptoms cause clinically significant distress or impairment in social, occupational, or other important areas of functioning.
- The disturbance is not attributable to the physiological effects of a substance (e.g., a drug of abuse, a medication) or another medical condition (e.g., hyperthyroidism).
- The disturbance is not better explained by another mental disorder (e.g., anxiety or worry about having panic attacks in panic disorder, negative evaluation in social anxiety disorder, contamination or other obsessions in obsessive-compulsive disorder, separation from attachment figures in separation anxiety disorder, reminders of traumatic events in posttraumatic stress disorder, gaining weight in anorexia nervosa, physical complaints in somatic symptom disorder, perceived appearance flaws in body dysmorphic disorder, having a serious illness in illness anxiety disorder, or the content

of delusional beliefs in schizophrenia or delusional disorder).

Case Study

Case Study: Sarah

Sarah is a 35-year-old woman who has been experiencing chronic and excessive worry for the past two years. Her anxiety is pervasive and affects various aspects of her life, including her job, relationships, and daily activities. Sarah's worry is disproportionate to the situations she encounters and is difficult for her to control. She often worries about her performance at work, her family's well-being, and potential negative events that may occur in the future.

Sarah's symptoms include:

- **Restlessness:** Sarah often feels on edge and finds it difficult to relax. She describes a constant sense of unease, as if something bad is about to happen.
- **Fatigue:** Despite getting adequate sleep, Sarah feels fatigued most of the time. Her constant worry drains her energy, leaving her feeling exhausted.
- **Difficulty Concentrating:** Sarah has trouble focusing on tasks at work and finds her mind frequently wandering to her worries. She often feels mentally foggy and has difficulty completing projects.
- **Irritability:** Sarah becomes easily irritated and snaps at her family and colleagues over minor issues. She

recognizes that her reactions are excessive but feels unable to control her irritability.

- **Muscle Tension:** Sarah experiences frequent muscle tension, particularly in her neck and shoulders. She often has headaches and finds herself clenching her jaw.
- **Sleep Disturbance:** Sarah has difficulty falling asleep due to racing thoughts and wakes up multiple times during the night. Her sleep is restless and unsatisfying, leaving her feeling unrefreshed in the morning.

Sarah's constant worry and physical symptoms have significantly impacted her quality of life. She avoids social situations and has difficulty enjoying activities that she once found pleasurable. Her performance at work has declined, and she feels overwhelmed by her responsibilities.

Concerned about her well-being, Sarah sought help from a mental health professional. After a comprehensive assessment, she was diagnosed with Generalized Anxiety Disorder. Her treatment plan included a combination of cognitive-behavioral therapy (CBT) and medication. CBT helped Sarah identify and challenge her irrational thoughts and develop coping strategies to manage her anxiety. The medication helped reduce the physical symptoms of anxiety, such as muscle tension and sleep disturbances.

Over several months of treatment, Sarah experienced a significant reduction in her anxiety symptoms. She learned techniques to manage her worry and improve her concentration and sleep. Sarah's relationships and work performance also improved as she gained better control over her anxiety.

Sarah's case highlights the importance of recognizing the symptoms of Generalized Anxiety Disorder and seeking appropriate treatment. With effective intervention, individuals with GAD can learn to manage their anxiety and lead more fulfilling lives.

Obsessive-Compulsive and Related Disorders

Key Features

Obsessive-Compulsive and Related Disorders are characterized by the presence of obsessions and/or compulsions that are time-consuming and cause significant distress or impairment in social, occupational, or other important areas of functioning. This category includes disorders such as Obsessive-Compulsive Disorder (OCD), Body Dysmorphic Disorder, Hoarding Disorder, Trichotillomania (Hair-Pulling Disorder), and Excoriation (Skin-Picking) Disorder.

Simplified Diagnostic Criteria

1. Obsessive-Compulsive Disorder (OCD)

- **Presence of obsessions, compulsions, or both**:
  - **Obsessions** are defined by (1) and (2):
    1. Recurrent and persistent thoughts, urges, or images that are experienced, at some

time during the disturbance, as intrusive and unwanted, and that in most individuals cause marked anxiety or distress.

2. The individual attempts to ignore or suppress such thoughts, urges, or images, or to neutralize them with some other thought or action (i.e., by performing a compulsion).

- o **Compulsions** are defined by (1) and (2):
  1. Repetitive behaviors (e.g., hand washing, ordering, checking) or mental acts (e.g., praying, counting, repeating words silently) that the individual feels driven to perform in response to an obsession, or according to rules that must be applied rigidly.
  2. The behaviors or mental acts are aimed at preventing or reducing anxiety or distress, or preventing some dreaded event or situation; however, these behaviors or mental acts are not connected in a realistic way with what they are designed to neutralize or prevent, or are clearly excessive.

- **The obsessions or compulsions are time-consuming** (e.g., take more than 1 hour per day) or cause clinically significant distress or impairment in social, occupational, or other important areas of functioning.

- **The obsessive-compulsive symptoms are not attributable to the physiological effects of a**

substance (e.g., a drug of abuse, a medication) or another medical condition.

- **The disturbance is not better explained by the symptoms of another mental disorder** (e.g., excessive worries, as in generalized anxiety disorder; preoccupation with appearance, as in body dysmorphic disorder; difficulty discarding or parting with possessions, as in hoarding disorder; hair pulling, as in trichotillomania [hair-pulling disorder]; skin picking, as in excoriation [skin-picking] disorder; stereotypies, as in stereotypic movement disorder; ritualized eating behavior, as in eating disorders; preoccupation with substances or gambling, as in substance-related and addictive disorders; preoccupation with having an illness, as in illness anxiety disorder; sexual urges or fantasies, as in paraphilic disorders; impulses, as in disruptive, impulse-control, and conduct disorders; guilty ruminations, as in major depressive disorder; thought insertion or delusional preoccupations, as in schizophrenia spectrum and other psychotic disorders; or repetitive patterns of behavior, as in autism spectrum disorder).

Case Study

Case Study: Mark

Mark is a 32-year-old man who has been struggling with obsessive-compulsive disorder (OCD) for over a decade. His daily life is severely impacted by persistent and intrusive thoughts that something terrible will happen if he doesn't perform certain rituals. Mark's obsessions are primarily centered around contamination and harm. He constantly fears that he or his loved ones will be contaminated by germs, leading to serious illness.

Mark's symptoms include:

- **Obsessions:** Mark experiences recurrent and intrusive thoughts about germs and contamination. He worries excessively that touching objects in public places will transfer deadly germs to his hands. These thoughts cause him significant anxiety and distress.
- **Compulsions:** To alleviate his anxiety, Mark engages in repetitive behaviors such as excessive hand washing, avoiding public places, and using hand sanitizers compulsively. He washes his hands dozens of times a day, sometimes for more than 30 minutes at a time, until his skin becomes raw and painful. Mark also avoids touching doorknobs, shaking hands, and using public restrooms.
- **Time-Consuming Rituals:** Mark's compulsive behaviors take up several hours of his day, interfering with his ability to work and maintain relationships. He is often late to appointments and avoids social interactions due to his rituals.
- **Impairment in Functioning:** Mark's OCD has significantly impaired his social and occupational functioning. He has difficulty concentrating at work because of his obsessive thoughts and feels embarrassed by his compulsions. His relationships with friends and

family have suffered because he avoids activities that might expose him to germs.

Mark's condition led him to seek help from a mental health professional. After a thorough assessment, he was diagnosed with Obsessive-Compulsive Disorder.

His treatment plan included a combination of cognitive-behavioral therapy (CBT) with an emphasis on exposure and response prevention (ERP) and medication. ERP helped Mark confront his fears and gradually reduce his compulsive behaviors. The medication helped alleviate some of his anxiety and made it easier for him to engage in therapy.

Through consistent therapy and support, Mark began to see improvements.

He learned to challenge his obsessive thoughts and reduce his compulsive behaviors. Although it was a gradual process, Mark was able to regain control over his life and reduce the impact of OCD on his daily functioning. He became more comfortable in social situations and was able to focus better at work.

Mark's case illustrates the significant impact that OCD can have on an individual's life and the importance of seeking appropriate treatment.

With effective intervention, individuals with OCD can learn to manage their symptoms and improve their quality of life.

Trauma and Stressor-Related Disorders

Key Features

Trauma and stressor-related disorders are characterized by exposure to a traumatic or stressful event and subsequent psychological distress. These disorders include Posttraumatic Stress Disorder (PTSD), Acute Stress Disorder, Adjustment Disorders, Reactive Attachment Disorder, and Disinhibited Social Engagement Disorder.

Symptoms can vary widely but generally include intrusive memories, avoidance behaviors, negative changes in thought and mood, and changes in physical and emotional reactions.

Simplified Diagnostic Criteria

1. Posttraumatic Stress Disorder (PTSD)

- **Exposure to actual or threatened death, serious injury, or sexual violence** in one (or more) of the following ways:
    1. Directly experiencing the traumatic event(s).
    2. Witnessing, in person, the event(s) as it occurred to others.
    3. Learning that the traumatic event(s) occurred to a close family member or close friend (cases of actual or threatened death must have been violent or accidental).

4. Experiencing repeated or extreme exposure to aversive details of the traumatic event(s) (e.g., first responders collecting human remains; police officers repeatedly exposed to details of child abuse).

- **Presence of one (or more) of the following intrusion symptoms** associated with the traumatic event(s), beginning after the traumatic event(s) occurred:
    1. Recurrent, involuntary, and intrusive distressing memories of the traumatic event(s).
    2. Recurrent distressing dreams in which the content and/or affect of the dream are related to the traumatic event(s).
    3. Dissociative reactions (e.g., flashbacks) in which the individual feels or acts as if the traumatic event(s) were recurring.
    4. Intense or prolonged psychological distress at exposure to internal or external cues that symbolize or resemble an aspect of the traumatic event(s).
    5. Marked physiological reactions to internal or external cues that symbolize or resemble an aspect of the traumatic event(s).
- **Persistent avoidance of stimuli associated with the traumatic event(s)**, beginning after the traumatic event(s) occurred, as evidenced by one or both of the following:
    1. Avoidance of or efforts to avoid distressing memories, thoughts, or feelings about or closely associated with the traumatic event(s).

2. Avoidance of or efforts to avoid external reminders (people, places, conversations, activities, objects, situations) that arouse distressing memories, thoughts, or feelings about or closely associated with the traumatic event(s).

- **Negative alterations in cognitions and mood associated with the traumatic event(s)**, beginning or worsening after the traumatic event(s) occurred, as evidenced by two (or more) of the following:
    1. Inability to remember an important aspect of the traumatic event(s) (typically due to dissociative amnesia and not to other factors such as head injury, alcohol, or drugs).
    2. Persistent and exaggerated negative beliefs or expectations about oneself, others, or the world (e.g., "I am bad," "No one can be trusted," "The world is completely dangerous").
    3. Persistent, distorted cognitions about the cause or consequences of the traumatic event(s) that lead the individual to blame himself/herself or others.
    4. Persistent negative emotional state (e.g., fear, horror, anger, guilt, or shame).
    5. Markedly diminished interest or participation in significant activities.
    6. Feelings of detachment or estrangement from others.
    7. Persistent inability to experience positive emotions (e.g., inability to experience happiness, satisfaction, or loving feelings).

- **Marked alterations in arousal and reactivity associated with the traumatic event(s)**, beginning or worsening after the traumatic event(s) occurred, as evidenced by two (or more) of the following:
  1. Irritable behavior and angry outbursts (with little or no provocation) typically expressed as verbal or physical aggression toward people or objects.
  2. Reckless or self-destructive behavior.
  3. Hypervigilance.
  4. Exaggerated startle response.
  5. Problems with concentration.
  6. Sleep disturbance (e.g., difficulty falling or staying asleep or restless sleep).
- **Duration of the disturbance (Criteria B, C, D, and E) is more than 1 month.**
- **The disturbance causes clinically significant distress or impairment** in social, occupational, or other important areas of functioning.
- **The disturbance is not attributable to the physiological effects of a substance** (e.g., medication, alcohol) or another medical condition.

Case Study

Case Study: David

David is a 40-year-old military veteran who served in combat zones for several years. Since returning home, he has been struggling with severe psychological distress. David experiences frequent flashbacks and nightmares related to his combat experiences, often waking up in a state of panic. He avoids activities and places that remind him of his service, such as fireworks displays, which resemble gunfire.

David's symptoms include:

- **Intrusive Memories:** David has recurrent and intrusive memories of the traumatic events he experienced during combat. These memories are vivid and distressing, often causing him to relive the events as if they were happening again.
- **Nightmares:** He suffers from distressing dreams in which he re-experiences the traumatic events. These nightmares disrupt his sleep, leaving him exhausted and on edge.
- **Avoidance:** David avoids talking about his military service and steers clear of situations that remind him of combat. He has stopped watching war movies and avoids public events where there are loud noises.
- **Negative Thoughts and Mood:** David feels a pervasive sense of guilt and shame, blaming himself for the deaths of fellow soldiers. He has lost interest in activities he once enjoyed and feels detached from his family and friends. He struggles to experience positive emotions and often feels numb.
- **Hyperarousal:** David is constantly on high alert, easily startled by sudden noises, and has difficulty concentrating. He is irritable and prone to angry outbursts, often over minor issues. His hypervigilance makes it hard for him to relax and feel safe.

David's condition led him to seek help from a mental health professional. After a thorough evaluation, he was diagnosed with Posttraumatic Stress Disorder (PTSD). His treatment plan included trauma-focused cognitive-behavioral therapy (CBT) and eye movement desensitization and reprocessing (EMDR) therapy. These therapies helped David process his traumatic memories and reduce his distress.

In addition to therapy, David was prescribed medication to manage his anxiety and improve his sleep. With ongoing treatment and support from his therapist and family, David began to see improvements in his symptoms. He learned coping strategies to manage his intrusive memories and hyperarousal and started to re-engage in activities he once enjoyed.

David's case highlights the significant impact of PTSD on an individual's life and the importance of seeking appropriate treatment. With effective intervention, individuals with PTSD can learn to manage their symptoms and improve their quality of life.

Dissociative Disorders

Key Features

Dissociative disorders are characterized by a disruption in the normal integration of consciousness, memory, identity, emotion, perception, body representation, motor control, and behavior. This category includes Dissociative Identity

Disorder (DID), Dissociative Amnesia, and Depersonalization/Derealization Disorder. These disruptions can cause significant distress or impairment in social, occupational, or other important areas of functioning.

Simplified Diagnostic Criteria

1. Dissociative Identity Disorder (DID)

- **Disruption of identity characterized by two or more distinct personality states,** which may be described in some cultures as an experience of possession. This disruption involves marked discontinuity in sense of self and sense of agency, accompanied by related alterations in affect, behavior, consciousness, memory, perception, cognition, and/or sensory-motor functioning. These signs and symptoms may be observed by others or reported by the individual.
- **Recurrent gaps in the recall of everyday events,** important personal information, and/or traumatic events that are inconsistent with ordinary forgetting.
- **The symptoms cause clinically significant distress or impairment** in social, occupational, or other important areas of functioning.
- **The disturbance is not a normal part of a broadly accepted cultural or religious practice.** (Note: In children, the symptoms are not better explained by imaginary playmates or other fantasy play.)

- **The symptoms are not attributable to the physiological effects of a substance** (e.g., blackouts or chaotic behavior during alcohol intoxication) or another medical condition (e.g., complex partial seizures).

2. Dissociative Amnesia

- **An inability to recall important autobiographical information**, usually of a traumatic or stressful nature, that is inconsistent with ordinary forgetting. Dissociative amnesia may be:
  - **Localized:** Inability to recall events during a specific period of time.
  - **Selective:** Inability to recall some, but not all, events during a specific period of time.
  - **Generalized:** Complete loss of memory for one's life history.
- **The symptoms cause clinically significant distress or impairment** in social, occupational, or other important areas of functioning.
- **The disturbance is not attributable to the physiological effects of a substance** (e.g., alcohol or other drug abuse, a medication) or a neurological or other medical condition (e.g., partial complex seizures, transient global amnesia).
- **The disturbance is not better explained by another mental disorder**, such as posttraumatic stress disorder, acute stress disorder, somatic symptom disorder, or major or mild neurocognitive disorder.

3. Depersonalization/Derealization Disorder

- **Presence of persistent or recurrent experiences of depersonalization, derealization, or both:**
    - **Depersonalization:** Experiences of unreality, detachment, or being an outside observer with respect to one's thoughts, feelings, sensations, body, or actions (e.g., perceptual alterations, distorted sense of time, unreal or absent self, emotional and/or physical numbing).
    - **Derealization:** Experiences of unreality or detachment with respect to surroundings (e.g., individuals or objects are experienced as unreal, dreamlike, foggy, lifeless, or visually distorted).
- **During the depersonalization or derealization experiences**, reality testing remains intact.
- **The symptoms cause clinically significant distress or impairment** in social, occupational, or other important areas of functioning.
- **The disturbance is not attributable to the physiological effects of a substance** (e.g., a drug of abuse, medication, or another medical condition, such as seizures).
- **The disturbance is not better explained by another mental disorder**, such as schizophrenia, panic disorder, major depressive disorder, acute stress disorder, posttraumatic stress disorder, or another dissociative disorder.

Case Study

Case Study: Lisa

Lisa is a 29-year-old woman who has been experiencing episodes of memory loss and changes in behavior for several years. She reports frequent gaps in her memory for daily activities and important events, such as not remembering significant conversations or activities with her family. Lisa's husband has noticed marked changes in her personality during these episodes, describing her as behaving like a different person with different tastes and preferences.

Lisa's symptoms include:

- **Disruption of Identity:** Lisa experiences distinct shifts in her personality, often feeling as though she is a different person. During these shifts, her voice, mannerisms, and preferences change significantly. For example, she may switch from being calm and introverted to outgoing and assertive without any apparent trigger.
- **Memory Gaps:** Lisa has recurrent gaps in her memory for everyday events and important personal information. She often forgets conversations, appointments, and even entire days. These memory gaps cause significant distress and confusion for both Lisa and her family.
- **Distress and Impairment:** Lisa's symptoms cause considerable distress and impair her ability to function in daily life. Her inconsistent behavior and memory problems have led to difficulties at work and strain in her

relationships. She often feels detached from herself and struggles to maintain a coherent sense of identity.

- **Cultural Considerations:** Lisa's symptoms are not part of any cultural or religious practice. Her experiences of identity disruption and memory loss are not consistent with cultural norms or traditions.

Concerned about her well-being, Lisa sought help from a mental health professional. After a comprehensive evaluation, including interviews and psychological assessments, she was diagnosed with Dissociative Identity Disorder (DID). Her treatment plan included psychotherapy, specifically trauma-focused therapy, to help her understand and integrate her different personality states. Lisa also began working on coping strategies to manage her memory gaps and reduce distress.

Through consistent therapy, Lisa started to gain insight into her condition and learn techniques to integrate her different identities. Her therapist helped her explore traumatic events from her past that may have contributed to her dissociation. Over time, Lisa made significant progress in understanding her experiences and improving her ability to function in daily life.

In addition to psychotherapy, Lisa also engaged in cognitive-behavioral therapy (CBT) to address any co-occurring anxiety and depression symptoms.

The combination of trauma-focused therapy and CBT helped Lisa develop a more stable sense of self and improve her overall mental health.

Extended Case Study: Dissociative Amnesia

Case Study: John

John is a 38-year-old man who was found wandering in a park with no recollection of how he got there or any details about his identity. When approached by the authorities, he could not provide any personal information, including his name, address, or details about his past. John was taken to a local hospital for evaluation.

John's symptoms include:

- **Localized Amnesia:** John has an inability to recall events that occurred over the past few days leading up to his being found in the park. He cannot remember significant personal information or recent events.
- **Generalized Amnesia:** After further evaluation, it was discovered that John has a complete loss of memory for his life history. He cannot recall any personal details, including his name, family, or past experiences.
- **Distress and Impairment:** John's inability to recall personal information causes him significant distress. He feels lost and disoriented, struggling to make sense of his surroundings and interactions with others.

Medical tests ruled out neurological conditions, substance use, and other medical causes for John's amnesia. A mental health professional was consulted, and after a thorough assessment, John was diagnosed with Dissociative Amnesia. His treatment plan included supportive therapy to help him feel safe and oriented, as well as techniques to gradually recover his lost memories. Over several weeks of therapy, John began to recall fragments of his past. His therapist used techniques such as hypnosis and guided imagery to help facilitate memory recovery. As John's memories started to return, he worked on integrating these experiences and understanding the possible psychological factors contributing to his amnesia.

John's case illustrates the severe impact that dissociative amnesia can have on an individual's life and the importance of seeking appropriate treatment. With effective intervention, individuals with dissociative amnesia can recover their memories and regain a sense of identity.

Somatic Symptom and Related Disorders

Key Features

Somatic symptom and related disorders are characterized by prominent somatic symptoms that are associated with significant distress and impairment. These disorders include Somatic Symptom Disorder, Illness Anxiety Disorder, Conversion Disorder (Functional Neurological Symptom Disorder), Factitious Disorder, and Psychological Factors

Affecting Other Medical Conditions. Individuals with these disorders often present with physical symptoms that cannot be fully explained by a general medical condition, substance use, or another mental disorder. The distress and impairment associated with these disorders can be severe, often leading individuals to seek extensive medical care.

Simplified Diagnostic Criteria

1. Somatic Symptom Disorder

- **One or more somatic symptoms that are distressing or result in significant disruption of daily life.**
- **Excessive thoughts, feelings, or behaviors related to the somatic symptoms or associated health concerns** as manifested by at least one of the following:
    1. Disproportionate and persistent thoughts about the seriousness of one's symptoms.
    2. Persistently high level of anxiety about health or symptoms.
    3. Excessive time and energy devoted to these symptoms or health concerns.
- **Although any one somatic symptom may not be continuously present, the state of being symptomatic is persistent** (typically more than 6 months).

2. Illness Anxiety Disorder

- **Preoccupation with having or acquiring a serious illness.**

- **Somatic symptoms are not present** or, if present, are only mild in intensity. If another medical condition is present or there is a high risk for developing a medical condition (e.g., strong family history is present), the preoccupation is clearly excessive or disproportionate.
- **There is a high level of anxiety about health**, and the individual is easily alarmed about personal health status.
- **The individual performs excessive health-related behaviors** (e.g., repeatedly checks his or her body for signs of illness) or exhibits maladaptive avoidance (e.g., avoids doctor appointments and hospitals).
- **Illness preoccupation has been present for at least 6 months**, but the specific illness that is feared may change over that period of time.
- **The illness-related preoccupation is not better explained by another mental disorder**, such as somatic symptom disorder, panic disorder, generalized anxiety disorder, obsessive-compulsive disorder, or delusional disorder, somatic type.

3. Conversion Disorder (Functional Neurological Symptom Disorder)

- **One or more symptoms of altered voluntary motor or sensory function.**
- **Clinical findings provide evidence of incompatibility** between the symptom and recognized neurological or medical conditions.
- **The symptom or deficit is not better explained by another medical or mental disorder.**

- **The symptom or deficit causes clinically significant distress or impairment** in social, occupational, or other important areas of functioning or warrants medical evaluation.

4. Factitious Disorder

- **Falsification of physical or psychological signs or symptoms**, or induction of injury or disease, associated with identified deception.
- **The individual presents himself or herself to others as ill, impaired, or injured.**
- **The deceptive behavior is evident** even in the absence of obvious external rewards.
- **The behavior is not better explained by another mental disorder**, such as delusional disorder or another psychotic disorder.

Case Study

Case Study: Mary

Mary is a 45-year-old woman who has been experiencing chronic pain and fatigue for several years. She frequently visits various doctors and specialists, seeking answers and relief for her symptoms. Despite extensive medical evaluations and tests, no clear medical cause has been identified. Mary's persistent physical symptoms have led to significant distress and impairment in her daily life.

Mary's symptoms include:

- **Chronic Pain:** Mary experiences ongoing pain in multiple areas of her body, including her back, neck, and joints. The pain is severe and affects her ability to perform daily activities.
- **Fatigue:** She often feels extremely tired and lacks the energy to engage in her usual routines. Simple tasks, such as getting out of bed and doing household chores, feel overwhelming.
- **Health Anxiety:** Mary is preoccupied with her health and constantly worries about the seriousness of her symptoms. She frequently searches for information online about possible medical conditions and believes that her symptoms are indicative of a serious illness.
- **Excessive Medical Visits:** Despite reassurances from multiple healthcare providers that her symptoms do not indicate a severe medical condition, Mary continues to seek further evaluations and treatments. She has undergone numerous tests and procedures, often with negative or inconclusive results.
- **Significant Disruption:** Mary's condition has led to significant disruption in her social and occupational life. She has difficulty maintaining relationships and has had to take a leave of absence from work due to her symptoms. Her constant preoccupation with her health prevents her from engaging in activities she once enjoyed.

Mary's condition led her to seek help from a mental health professional. After a thorough assessment, she was diagnosed with Somatic Symptom Disorder. Her treatment plan included cognitive-behavioral therapy (CBT) to help her address her excessive health-related thoughts and behaviors. CBT provided Mary with strategies to manage her anxiety and reduce her preoccupation with her symptoms. Techniques such as cognitive restructuring helped her challenge and change her disproportionate thoughts about the seriousness of her symptoms.

Mary also participated in mindfulness-based stress reduction (MBSR) to help her manage her physical symptoms and improve her overall well-being. MBSR taught Mary techniques to focus on the present moment and reduce the impact of her somatic symptoms on her daily life.

Through therapy, Mary began to understand the connection between her physical symptoms and psychological factors. She learned techniques to manage her pain and improve her coping skills. Although her physical symptoms did not completely disappear, Mary experienced a significant reduction in her distress and was able to regain some control over her life. She started to re-engage in social activities and gradually returned to work.

Mary's case highlights the importance of recognizing the role of psychological factors in somatic symptom disorders and seeking appropriate treatment. With effective intervention, individuals with Somatic Symptom Disorder can learn to manage their symptoms and improve their quality of life. Mary's progress demonstrates how a comprehensive treatment approach that includes both psychological and medical interventions can help individuals achieve better outcomes.

Feeding and Eating Disorders

Key Features

Feeding and eating disorders are characterized by persistent disturbances of eating or eating-related behavior that result in the altered consumption or absorption of food and significantly impair physical health or psychosocial functioning. This category includes disorders such as Anorexia Nervosa, Bulimia Nervosa, Binge-Eating Disorder, Pica, and Rumination Disorder. These disorders can have severe physical and psychological consequences if not properly treated.

Simplified Diagnostic Criteria

1. Anorexia Nervosa

- **Restriction of energy intake relative to requirements**, leading to a significantly low body weight in the context of age, sex, developmental trajectory, and physical health. Significantly low weight is defined as a weight that is less than minimally normal or, for children and adolescents, less than that minimally expected.

- **Intense fear of gaining weight or becoming fat**, or persistent behavior that interferes with weight gain, even though at a significantly low weight.
- **Disturbance in the way in which one's body weight or shape is experienced**, undue influence of body weight or shape on self-evaluation, or persistent lack of recognition of the seriousness of the current low body weight.

2. Bulimia Nervosa

- **Recurrent episodes of binge eating**, characterized by both of the following:
    1. Eating, in a discrete period of time (e.g., within any 2-hour period), an amount of food that is definitely larger than what most people would eat in a similar period of time under similar circumstances.
    2. A sense of lack of control over eating during the episode (e.g., a feeling that one cannot stop eating or control what or how much one is eating).
- **Recurrent inappropriate compensatory behaviors** in order to prevent weight gain, such as self-induced vomiting, misuse of laxatives, diuretics, or other medications, fasting, or excessive exercise.
- **The binge eating and inappropriate compensatory behaviors both occur**, on average, at least once a week for 3 months.
- **Self-evaluation is unduly influenced by body shape and weight.**

- **The disturbance does not occur exclusively during episodes of Anorexia Nervosa.**

3. Binge-Eating Disorder

- **Recurrent episodes of binge eating**, as characterized by both:
  1. Eating, in a discrete period of time (e.g., within any 2-hour period), an amount of food that is definitely larger than what most people would eat in a similar period of time under similar circumstances.
  2. A sense of lack of control over eating during the episode.
- **Binge-eating episodes are associated with three (or more) of the following:**
  1. Eating much more rapidly than normal.
  2. Eating until feeling uncomfortably full.
  3. Eating large amounts of food when not feeling physically hungry.
  4. Eating alone because of feeling embarrassed by how much one is eating.
  5. Feeling disgusted with oneself, depressed, or very guilty afterward.
- **Marked distress regarding binge eating is present.**
- **The binge eating occurs**, on average, at least once a week for 3 months.
- **The binge eating is not associated with the recurrent use of inappropriate compensatory behavior** as in

bulimia nervosa and does not occur exclusively during the course of bulimia nervosa or anorexia nervosa.

Case Study

Case Study: Emma

Emma is a 17-year-old high school student who has been struggling with an intense fear of gaining weight. Over the past year, she has significantly restricted her food intake, resulting in a noticeable weight loss. Emma's parents became concerned when they noticed her dramatic weight loss and changes in her eating habits. Despite being underweight, Emma insists that she is "too fat" and is obsessed with losing more weight.

Emma's symptoms include:

- **Restriction of Food Intake:** Emma eats very little, often skipping meals and consuming only small portions of low-calorie foods. She meticulously counts calories and avoids foods she perceives as fattening.
- **Intense Fear of Gaining Weight:** Emma is terrified of gaining weight and engages in behaviors aimed at preventing weight gain, such as excessive exercise and avoiding social situations where food is involved.
- **Body Image Disturbance:** Emma perceives herself as overweight, despite being significantly underweight. She frequently checks her body in the mirror and is preoccupied with thoughts about her weight and body shape.

- **Physical Health Consequences:** Emma's severe weight loss has led to physical health problems, including fatigue, dizziness, and amenorrhea (loss of menstrual periods). Her energy levels are low, and she often feels weak.

Emma's condition led her parents to seek help from a mental health professional. After a comprehensive evaluation, Emma was diagnosed with Anorexia Nervosa. Her treatment plan included a multidisciplinary approach involving a therapist, dietitian, and physician. The goals of her treatment were to restore her weight, address her distorted thoughts about body image, and develop healthy eating behaviors.

Emma participated in cognitive-behavioral therapy (CBT) to challenge her irrational beliefs about weight and body image. She also worked with a dietitian to develop a balanced meal plan and gradually increase her food intake. Medical monitoring was essential to ensure her physical health was improving.

Through consistent treatment and support from her family, Emma began to make progress. She started to gain weight and improve her physical health. Therapy helped her develop a more positive body image and reduce her fear of weight gain. Although recovery was a gradual process, Emma learned coping strategies to manage her anxiety about food and body image.

Emma's case highlights the severe impact of Anorexia Nervosa on physical and mental health and the importance of early intervention and a comprehensive treatment approach. With appropriate treatment, individuals with Anorexia Nervosa can recover and regain a healthy relationship with food and their bodies.

Sleep-Wake Disorders

Key Features

Sleep-wake disorders involve problems with the quality, timing, and amount of sleep, which result in daytime distress and impairment in functioning. These disorders include Insomnia Disorder, Hypersomnolence Disorder, Narcolepsy, Obstructive Sleep Apnea Hypopnea, Circadian Rhythm Sleep-Wake Disorders, and Parasomnias. Proper diagnosis and treatment of these disorders are crucial for improving an individual's overall health and well-being.

Simplified Diagnostic Criteria

1. Insomnia Disorder

- **A predominant complaint of dissatisfaction with sleep quantity or quality**, associated with one (or more) of the following symptoms:
    1. Difficulty initiating sleep.
    2. Difficulty maintaining sleep, characterized by frequent awakenings or problems returning to sleep after awakenings.
    3. Early-morning awakening with an inability to return to sleep.

- The sleep disturbance causes clinically significant distress or impairment in social, occupational, educational, academic, behavioral, or other important areas of functioning.
- The sleep difficulty occurs at least 3 nights per week.
- The sleep difficulty is present for at least 3 months.
- The sleep difficulty occurs despite adequate opportunity for sleep.
- The insomnia is not better explained by and does not occur exclusively during the course of another sleep-wake disorder (e.g., narcolepsy, a breathing-related sleep disorder, a circadian rhythm sleep-wake disorder, a parasomnia).
- The insomnia is not attributable to the physiological effects of a substance (e.g., a drug of abuse, a medication).
- Coexisting mental disorders and medical conditions do not adequately explain the predominant complaint of insomnia.

2. Hypersomnolence Disorder

- Self-reported excessive sleepiness (hypersomnolence) despite a main sleep period lasting at least 7 hours, with at least one of the following symptoms:
    1. Recurrent periods of sleep or lapses into sleep within the same day.

2. A prolonged main sleep episode of more than 9 hours per day that is nonrestorative (i.e., unrefreshing).

3. Difficulty being fully awake after abrupt awakening.

- **The hypersomnolence occurs at least three times per week,** for at least 3 months.
- **The hypersomnolence is accompanied by significant distress or impairment** in cognitive, social, occupational, or other important areas of functioning.
- **The hypersomnolence is not better explained by and does not occur exclusively during the course of another sleep disorder.**
- **The hypersomnolence is not attributable to the physiological effects of a substance** (e.g., a drug of abuse, a medication).
- **Coexisting mental and medical disorders do not adequately explain the predominant complaint of hypersomnolence.**

Case Study

Case Study: James

James is a 35-year-old software engineer who has been experiencing severe difficulties with sleep for the past year. Despite feeling exhausted, James struggles to fall asleep at night and often wakes up multiple times throughout the night. He reports waking up too early in the morning and being unable to return to sleep, leaving him feeling fatigued and irritable during the day.

James's symptoms include:

- **Difficulty Initiating Sleep:** James finds it hard to fall asleep, often lying awake for hours despite feeling tired.
- **Frequent Awakenings:** He wakes up several times during the night and has trouble falling back asleep.
- **Early-Morning Awakening:** James wakes up much earlier than he needs to and cannot return to sleep, resulting in insufficient sleep duration.
- **Daytime Fatigue:** Due to his poor sleep quality, James feels constantly tired during the day, which affects his performance at work and his ability to concentrate.
- **Impairment in Daily Functioning:** His lack of sleep leads to irritability and difficulty in maintaining social relationships. He often feels too tired to engage in activities he once enjoyed.

Concerned about his persistent sleep problems, James sought help from a sleep specialist. After a thorough evaluation, including a sleep diary and polysomnography (sleep study), James was diagnosed with Insomnia Disorder. His treatment plan included cognitive-behavioral therapy for insomnia (CBT-I), which focused on changing his sleep habits and addressing any negative thoughts and behaviors that were contributing to his insomnia.

CBT-I helped James establish a consistent sleep schedule, reduce the time spent in bed awake, and create a relaxing bedtime routine. He also learned techniques to manage stress and anxiety that were interfering with his sleep. Additionally, his sleep specialist recommended some lifestyle changes, such as reducing caffeine intake and avoiding electronic devices before bedtime.

Through consistent application of these strategies, James began to see improvements in his sleep. He was able to fall asleep more quickly, stay asleep longer, and wake up feeling more refreshed. His daytime functioning improved, and he felt more energetic and focused at work.

James's case highlights the importance of addressing insomnia and the effectiveness of CBT-I in treating this common sleep disorder. With appropriate intervention, individuals with insomnia can improve their sleep quality and overall well-being.

Sexual Dysfunctions

Key Features

Sexual dysfunctions involve a clinically significant disturbance in a person's ability to respond sexually or experience sexual pleasure. These disorders can cause significant distress and interpersonal difficulties. Sexual dysfunctions include Delayed Ejaculation, Erectile Disorder, Female Orgasmic Disorder, Female Sexual Interest/Arousal Disorder, Genito-Pelvic Pain/Penetration Disorder, Male Hypoactive Sexual Desire Disorder, Premature (Early)

Ejaculation, and Substance/Medication-Induced Sexual Dysfunction.

Simplified Diagnostic Criteria

1. Erectile Disorder

- **At least one of the following symptoms must be experienced** on almost all or all (approximately 75%-100%) occasions of sexual activity (in identified situational contexts or, if generalized, in all contexts):
  1. Marked difficulty in obtaining an erection during sexual activity.
  2. Marked difficulty in maintaining an erection until the completion of sexual activity.
  3. Marked decrease in erectile rigidity.
- **The symptoms in Criterion A have persisted for a minimum duration of approximately 6 months.**
- **The symptoms cause clinically significant distress** in the individual.
- **The sexual dysfunction is not better explained by a nonsexual mental disorder** or as a consequence of severe relationship distress or other significant stressors and is not attributable to the effects of a substance/medication or another medical condition.

2. Female Sexual Interest/Arousal Disorder

- **Lack of, or significantly reduced, sexual interest/arousal**, as manifested by at least three of the following:

1. Absent/reduced interest in sexual activity.
2. Absent/reduced sexual/erotic thoughts or fantasies.
3. No/reduced initiation of sexual activity, and typically unreceptive to a partner's attempts to initiate.
4. Absent/reduced sexual excitement/pleasure during sexual activity in almost all or all (approximately 75%-100%) sexual encounters.
5. Absent/reduced sexual interest/arousal in response to any internal or external sexual/erotic cues (e.g., written, verbal, visual).
6. Absent/reduced genital or nongenital sensations during sexual activity in almost all or all (approximately 75%-100%) sexual encounters.

- **The symptoms in Criterion A have persisted for a minimum duration of approximately 6 months.**
- **The symptoms cause clinically significant distress** in the individual.
- **The sexual dysfunction is not better explained by a nonsexual mental disorder** or as a consequence of severe relationship distress or other significant stressors and is not attributable to the effects of a substance/medication or another medical condition.

3. Premature (Early) Ejaculation

- **A persistent or recurrent pattern of ejaculation occurring during partnered sexual activity within**

approximately 1 minute following vaginal penetration and before the individual wishes it.

- **The symptoms in Criterion A must have been present for at least 6 months** and must be experienced on almost all or all (approximately 75%-100%) occasions of sexual activity (in identified situational contexts or, if generalized, in all contexts).
- **The symptoms cause clinically significant distress** in the individual.
- **The sexual dysfunction is not better explained by a nonsexual mental disorder** or as a consequence of severe relationship distress or other significant stressors and is not attributable to the effects of a substance/medication or another medical condition.

Case Study

Case Study: John

John is a 45-year-old man who has been experiencing difficulties with achieving and maintaining an erection during sexual activity for the past year.

This issue has caused significant distress for him and has affected his relationship with his partner. John reports that his confidence and self-esteem have been impacted, and he feels anxious about engaging in sexual activity.

John's symptoms include:

- **Difficulty Obtaining an Erection:** John struggles to achieve an erection despite feeling sexually aroused. This issue occurs consistently during sexual activity.
- **Difficulty Maintaining an Erection:** Even when John manages to achieve an erection, he finds it challenging to maintain it until the completion of sexual activity.
- **Decreased Erectile Rigidity:** John notices that his erections are not as firm as they used to be, which further contributes to his distress and anxiety.

John's condition led him to seek help from a urologist, who conducted a thorough medical evaluation to rule out any underlying medical conditions. The evaluation included a physical examination, blood tests, and assessments of his hormone levels. After ruling out physical causes, John was referred to a mental health professional for further evaluation.

During the assessment, John disclosed that he had been experiencing significant work-related stress and was feeling overwhelmed by his responsibilities. He also reported that his relationship with his partner had been strained due to his erectile difficulties, which added to his anxiety. Based on the assessment, John was diagnosed with Erectile Disorder.

John's treatment plan included a combination of psychological and medical interventions. He was prescribed a medication to help improve his erectile function and was also referred to a therapist for cognitive-behavioral therapy

(CBT). CBT helped John address his anxiety and negative thoughts related to sexual performance. He learned relaxation techniques and strategies to reduce his stress levels.

Through therapy, John also worked on improving communication with his partner about his condition. This helped reduce the pressure he felt and fostered a supportive environment. Over time, John noticed improvements in his erectile function and overall sexual satisfaction.

John's case highlights the importance of addressing both the psychological and physical aspects of sexual dysfunction. With appropriate treatment and support, individuals with Erectile Disorder can experience significant improvements in their sexual health and relationships.

Disruptive, Impulse-Control, and Conduct Disorders

Key Features

Disruptive, impulse-control, and conduct disorders involve problems in the self-control of emotions and behaviors. These problems often manifest in behaviors that violate the rights of others (e.g., aggression, destruction of property) and/or bring the individual into significant conflict with societal norms or authority figures. This category includes Oppositional Defiant Disorder (ODD), Intermittent

Explosive Disorder, Conduct Disorder, Antisocial Personality Disorder, Pyromania, and Kleptomania.

Simplified Diagnostic Criteria

1. Oppositional Defiant Disorder (ODD)

- **A pattern of angry/irritable mood, argumentative/defiant behavior, or vindictiveness lasting at least 6 months,** as evidenced by at least four symptoms from any of the following categories, and exhibited during interaction with at least one individual who is not a sibling:
  - **Angry/Irritable Mood:**
    1. Often loses temper.
    2. Is often touchy or easily annoyed.
    3. Is often angry and resentful.
  - **Argumentative/Defiant Behavior:**
    1. Often argues with authority figures or, for children and adolescents, with adults.
    2. Often actively defies or refuses to comply with requests from authority figures or with rules.
    3. Often deliberately annoys others.
    4. Often blames others for his or her mistakes or misbehavior.
  - **Vindictiveness:**
    1. Has been spiteful or vindictive at least twice within the past 6 months.

- **The disturbance in behavior is associated with distress in the individual or others in his or her immediate social context** (e.g., family, peer group, work colleagues), or it impacts negatively on social, educational, occupational, or other important areas of functioning.
- **The behaviors do not occur exclusively during the course of a psychotic, substance use, depressive, or bipolar disorder.** Also, the criteria are not met for disruptive mood dysregulation disorder.

2. Conduct Disorder

- **A repetitive and persistent pattern of behavior in which the basic rights of others or major age-appropriate societal norms or rules are violated,** as manifested by the presence of at least three of the following 15 criteria in the past 12 months from any of the categories below, with at least one criterion present in the past 6 months:
  - **Aggression to People and Animals:**
    1. Often bullies, threatens, or intimidates others.
    2. Often initiates physical fights.
    3. Has used a weapon that can cause serious physical harm to others (e.g., a bat, brick, broken bottle, knife, gun).
    4. Has been physically cruel to people.
    5. Has been physically cruel to animals.

6. Has stolen while confronting a victim (e.g., mugging, purse snatching, extortion, armed robbery).

7. Has forced someone into sexual activity.

o **Destruction of Property**:

1. Has deliberately engaged in fire setting with the intention of causing serious damage.

2. Has deliberately destroyed others' property (other than by fire setting).

o **Deceitfulness or Theft**:

1. Has broken into someone else's house, building, or car.

2. Often lies to obtain goods or favors or to avoid obligations (i.e., "cons" others).

3. Has stolen items of nontrivial value without confronting a victim (e.g., shoplifting, but without breaking and entering; forgery).

o **Serious Violations of Rules**:

1. Often stays out at night despite parental prohibitions, beginning before age 13 years.

2. Has run away from home overnight at least twice while living in the parental or parental surrogate home (or once without returning for a lengthy period).

3. Is often truant from school, beginning before age 13 years.

- **The disturbance in behavior causes clinically significant impairment** in social, academic, or occupational functioning.
- **If the individual is age 18 years or older, criteria are not met for antisocial personality disorder.**

Case Study

Case Study: Ethan

Ethan is a 15-year-old boy who has been displaying increasingly aggressive and defiant behavior over the past year. He frequently argues with his parents and teachers, deliberately breaks rules, and shows little regard for the rights of others. Ethan's parents became concerned when his behavior escalated to physical altercations with peers and vandalism in the community.

Ethan's symptoms include:

- **Aggression to People:** Ethan has been involved in multiple physical fights at school and has threatened classmates. He often initiates these confrontations and shows little remorse for his actions.
- **Destruction of Property:** He has been caught vandalizing school property and has set small fires in his neighborhood.
- **Deceitfulness:** Ethan frequently lies to his parents about his whereabouts and has stolen money from them on several occasions.

- **Serious Violations of Rules:** He often stays out late at night without permission and has been truant from school several times.

Ethan's behavior has resulted in several suspensions from school and increasing isolation from his peers. His academic performance has declined, and he has lost interest in activities he once enjoyed. His parents are struggling to manage his behavior and have sought help from a mental health professional.

After a comprehensive evaluation, Ethan was diagnosed with Conduct Disorder. His treatment plan included individual therapy to address his aggressive behavior and underlying emotional issues. He also participated in family therapy to improve communication and establish consistent rules and consequences at home.

Ethan's therapist used cognitive-behavioral techniques to help him develop better problem-solving skills and manage his anger. He also worked on building empathy and understanding the impact of his actions on others. Through consistent therapy and support from his family, Ethan began to show improvements. He became more aware of his behavior and started to make better choices.

Ethan's case highlights the importance of early intervention and comprehensive treatment for individuals with Conduct Disorder. With appropriate support and therapy, individuals with Conduct Disorder can learn to manage their behavior and improve their social and academic functioning.

Substance-Related and Addictive Disorders

Key Features

Substance-related and addictive disorders involve the excessive use of substances such as alcohol, tobacco, and drugs, leading to significant impairment or distress. These disorders also include behavioral addictions such as gambling disorder. The DSM-5-TR classifies these disorders based on the substance involved and the specific criteria related to the problematic use. The key features often include a strong desire to use the substance, difficulty controlling its use, and continued use despite harmful consequences.

Simplified Diagnostic Criteria

1. Alcohol Use Disorder

- **A problematic pattern of alcohol use leading to clinically significant impairment or distress**, as manifested by at least two of the following, occurring within a 12-month period:
    1. Alcohol is often taken in larger amounts or over a longer period than was intended.
    2. There is a persistent desire or unsuccessful efforts to cut down or control alcohol use.
    3. A great deal of time is spent in activities necessary to obtain alcohol, use alcohol, or recover from its effects.
    4. Craving, or a strong desire or urge to use alcohol.

5. Recurrent alcohol use resulting in a failure to fulfill major role obligations at work, school, or home.

6. Continued alcohol use despite having persistent or recurrent social or interpersonal problems caused or exacerbated by the effects of alcohol.

7. Important social, occupational, or recreational activities are given up or reduced because of alcohol use.

8. Recurrent alcohol use in situations in which it is physically hazardous.

9. Alcohol use is continued despite knowledge of having a persistent or recurrent physical or psychological problem that is likely to have been caused or exacerbated by alcohol.

10. Tolerance, as defined by either of the following:

   ▪ A need for markedly increased amounts of alcohol to achieve intoxication or desired effect.

   ▪ A markedly diminished effect with continued use of the same amount of alcohol.

11. Withdrawal, as manifested by either of the following:

   ▪ The characteristic withdrawal syndrome for alcohol.

   ▪ Alcohol (or a closely related substance, such as a benzodiazepine) is taken to relieve or avoid withdrawal symptoms.

2. Gambling Disorder

- **Persistent and recurrent problematic gambling behavior leading to clinically significant impairment or distress**, as indicated by the individual exhibiting four (or more) of the following in a 12-month period:

    1. Needs to gamble with increasing amounts of money to achieve the desired excitement.
    2. Is restless or irritable when attempting to cut down or stop gambling.
    3. Has made repeated unsuccessful efforts to control, cut back, or stop gambling.
    4. Is often preoccupied with gambling (e.g., having persistent thoughts of reliving past gambling experiences, handicapping or planning the next venture, thinking of ways to get money with which to gamble).
    5. Often gambles when feeling distressed (e.g., helpless, guilty, anxious, depressed).
    6. After losing money gambling, often returns another day to get even ("chasing" one's losses).
    7. Lies to conceal the extent of involvement with gambling.
    8. Has jeopardized or lost a significant relationship, job, or educational or career opportunity because of gambling.
    9. Relies on others to provide money to relieve desperate financial situations caused by gambling.

- **The gambling behavior is not better explained by a manic episode.**

Case Study

Case Study: Michael

Michael is a 42-year-old man who has been struggling with alcohol use for over a decade. He initially began drinking socially, but over the years, his alcohol consumption increased significantly. Michael's family and friends have expressed concern about his drinking, but he has been unable to cut down despite multiple attempts.

Michael's symptoms include:

- **Increased Consumption:** Michael often drinks larger amounts of alcohol than he intends. What starts as a single drink in the evening frequently turns into several drinks, lasting late into the night.
- **Failed Attempts to Cut Down:** Despite recognizing the negative impact of his drinking, Michael has made several unsuccessful attempts to reduce his alcohol intake. He experiences strong cravings and finds it difficult to resist the urge to drink.
- **Time Spent Drinking:** A significant portion of Michael's time is dedicated to drinking or recovering from its effects. He often misses family events and social activities because of his drinking.
- **Neglected Responsibilities:** Michael's alcohol use has led to frequent absences from work and deteriorating performance. He has missed important deadlines and meetings, jeopardizing his career.

- **Continued Use Despite Problems:** Michael continues to drink despite experiencing recurrent arguments with his spouse about his alcohol use and its impact on their relationship.
- **Tolerance and Withdrawal:** He needs to consume increasing amounts of alcohol to feel its effects and experiences withdrawal symptoms, such as tremors and anxiety, when he tries to stop drinking.

Concerned about his health and the strain on his relationships, Michael decided to seek help. He contacted a substance abuse counselor and began attending group therapy sessions. After a comprehensive assessment, Michael was diagnosed with Alcohol Use Disorder.

Michael's treatment plan included a combination of individual counseling, group therapy, and medication to help manage his withdrawal symptoms. He participated in cognitive-behavioral therapy (CBT) to address the underlying issues contributing to his alcohol use and to develop coping strategies for dealing with stress and cravings.

Through therapy, Michael learned to identify triggers for his drinking and developed healthier ways to manage stress. He also worked on repairing his relationships and rebuilding trust with his family. Over time, Michael's commitment to his recovery led to significant improvements. He reduced his alcohol consumption, improved his work performance, and reconnected with his loved ones.

Michael's case highlights the challenges of Alcohol Use Disorder and the importance of comprehensive treatment. With appropriate support and intervention, individuals struggling with substance use can achieve recovery and improve their quality of life.

Neurocognitive Disorders

Key Features

Neurocognitive disorders are characterized by a decline in cognitive functioning that is not attributable to normal aging. These disorders often affect memory, attention, learning, language, perception, and social cognition. The DSM-5-TR classifies neurocognitive disorders into major and mild categories based on the severity of the cognitive decline. These disorders include Alzheimer's disease, frontotemporal lobar degeneration, Lewy body disease, vascular disease, traumatic brain injury, substance/medication use, HIV infection, prion disease, Parkinson's disease, Huntington's disease, and other medical conditions.

Neurocognitive disorders can significantly impact an individual's ability to live independently, affecting their ability to perform everyday activities and maintain relationships. Early diagnosis and intervention are crucial in managing these disorders and improving the quality of life for affected individuals and their families.

Simplified Diagnostic Criteria
1. Major Neurocognitive Disorder (NCD)

- **Significant cognitive decline from a previous level of performance** in one or more cognitive domains (complex attention, executive function, learning and memory, language, perceptual-motor, or social cognition) based on:
  1. Concern of the individual, a knowledgeable informant, or the clinician that there has been a significant decline in cognitive function; and
  2. A substantial impairment in cognitive performance, preferably documented by standardized neuropsychological testing or, in its absence, another quantified clinical assessment.
- **The cognitive deficits interfere with independence in everyday activities** (i.e., at a minimum, requiring assistance with complex instrumental activities of daily living such as paying bills or managing medications).
- **The cognitive deficits do not occur exclusively in the context of delirium.**
- **The cognitive deficits are not better explained by another mental disorder** (e.g., major depressive disorder, schizophrenia).

2. Mild Neurocognitive Disorder (NCD)

- **Modest cognitive decline from a previous level of performance** in one or more cognitive domains (complex attention, executive function, learning and memory, language, perceptual-motor, or social cognition) based on:

1. Concern of the individual, a knowledgeable informant, or the clinician that there has been a mild decline in cognitive function; and
2. A modest impairment in cognitive performance, preferably documented by standardized neuropsychological testing or, in its absence, another quantified clinical assessment.

- **The cognitive deficits do not interfere with capacity for independence in everyday activities** (i.e., complex instrumental activities of daily living such as paying bills or managing medications are preserved, but greater effort, compensatory strategies, or accommodation may be required).
- **The cognitive deficits do not occur exclusively in the context of delirium.**
- **The cognitive deficits are not better explained by another mental disorder** (e.g., major depressive disorder, schizophrenia).

Types of Neurocognitive Disorders

1. Alzheimer's Disease

- **Most common cause of Major NCD.**
- **Gradual onset and continuing cognitive decline.**
- **Characterized by memory impairment, especially in learning new information, and one or more additional cognitive deficits (e.g., aphasia, apraxia, agnosia, or executive function disturbances).**

2. Vascular Neurocognitive Disorder

- Cognitive decline resulting from cerebrovascular disease.
- Typically characterized by a stepwise progression of symptoms.
- Symptoms may include impaired judgment, difficulty with decision-making, and planning.

3. Frontotemporal Neurocognitive Disorder

- Characterized by prominent changes in personality, behavior, and language.
- Often involves socially inappropriate behaviors, apathy, and language disturbances such as aphasia.

4. Lewy Body Dementia

- Fluctuating cognition, recurrent visual hallucinations, and motor symptoms similar to Parkinson's disease.
- May also include REM sleep behavior disorder and severe sensitivity to antipsychotic medications.

5. Traumatic Brain Injury (TBI)

- Cognitive impairments resulting from a head injury.
- Symptoms can include memory loss, attention deficits, impaired executive function, and emotional disturbances.

Case Study

Case Study: Mary

Mary is a 70-year-old retired school teacher who has been experiencing memory problems for the past two years. She often forgets recent conversations, misplaces items, and has difficulty finding the right words during conversations. Her family has also noticed that she has become more disoriented and confused, particularly when navigating familiar places.

Mary's symptoms include:

- **Memory Impairment:** Mary frequently forgets appointments and important dates. She often repeats questions and conversations because she cannot recall having them.
- **Language Difficulties:** She struggles to find the right words and often substitutes incorrect words during conversations.
- **Disorientation:** Mary becomes disoriented in familiar environments, sometimes getting lost while driving to routine destinations.
- **Impaired Daily Functioning:** Due to her cognitive decline, Mary has difficulty managing her finances and medications. She needs assistance from her family for these tasks.
- **Behavioral Changes:** Mary's family has also observed changes in her mood and behavior, including increased irritability and withdrawal from social activities.

Concerned about her declining cognitive abilities, Mary's family encouraged her to seek medical evaluation. After a comprehensive assessment, including neuropsychological testing and brain imaging, Mary was diagnosed with Major Neurocognitive Disorder due to Alzheimer's disease.

Mary's treatment plan included medications to manage symptoms and slow cognitive decline, such as cholinesterase inhibitors. She also participated in cognitive rehabilitation therapy to help improve her cognitive function and maintain independence in daily activities. Mary's family was involved in her care, providing support and assisting with tasks she found challenging.

In addition to medical and therapeutic interventions, Mary and her family received education about Alzheimer's disease and were connected with support groups to share experiences and resources. This comprehensive approach helped Mary manage her symptoms and maintain her quality of life.

Mary's family played a crucial role in her care. They adapted the home environment to ensure her safety, established a daily routine to provide structure, and engaged her in mentally stimulating activities to support cognitive function. They also took measures to address her behavioral changes, using techniques learned from support groups and healthcare providers.

Mary's case highlights the importance of early diagnosis and a multifaceted treatment approach for individuals with neurocognitive disorders. With appropriate interventions, individuals with Major Neurocognitive Disorder can receive the support they need to manage their symptoms and maintain their independence for as long as possible.

Extended Case Study: Vascular Neurocognitive Disorder

Case Study: Robert

Robert is a 68-year-old man who has a history of hypertension and diabetes. Over the past year, his family has noticed a decline in his cognitive abilities. He has become increasingly forgetful, has difficulty following instructions, and often struggles with decision-making. His family also reports that he has experienced several small strokes.

Robert's symptoms include:

- **Impaired Judgment:** Robert has difficulty making decisions, often struggling with tasks that require planning and organization.
- **Memory Loss:** He frequently forgets recent events and conversations, and has trouble recalling information he once knew well.
- **Behavioral Changes:** Robert has become more irritable and exhibits mood swings. His family has noticed that he often becomes frustrated easily.
- **Physical Symptoms:** Robert has experienced weakness on one side of his body and has difficulty with

coordination, likely due to the small strokes he has suffered.

Concerned about his cognitive and physical health, Robert's family took him to see a neurologist. After a comprehensive assessment, including a neurological exam, brain imaging, and cognitive testing, Robert was diagnosed with Major Neurocognitive Disorder due to Vascular Disease.

Robert's treatment plan included managing his vascular risk factors to prevent further strokes, such as controlling his blood pressure and blood sugar levels, adopting a heart-healthy diet, and engaging in regular physical activity. He was also prescribed medications to manage his cognitive symptoms and improve his quality of life.

Robert participated in cognitive rehabilitation to help improve his cognitive function and relearn skills affected by the strokes. His family was involved in his care, providing support with daily activities and helping to monitor his health. They also made modifications to their home to ensure his safety and support his independence.

Through a combination of medical management, cognitive rehabilitation, and family support, Robert was able to stabilize his condition and maintain a reasonable quality of life. His case highlights the importance of addressing underlying medical conditions in the management of neurocognitive disorders and the benefits of a comprehensive care approach.

Personality Disorders

Key Features

Personality disorders are characterized by enduring patterns of behavior, cognition, and inner experience that deviate markedly from the expectations of an individual's culture. These patterns are pervasive and inflexible, have an onset in adolescence or early adulthood, are stable over time, and lead to distress or impairment. The DSM-5-TR categorizes personality disorders into three clusters: Cluster A (odd or eccentric disorders), Cluster B (dramatic, emotional, or erratic disorders), and Cluster C (anxious or fearful disorders).

Simplified Diagnostic Criteria

1. Borderline Personality Disorder (BPD)

- **A pervasive pattern of instability of interpersonal relationships, self-image, and affects, and marked impulsivity,** beginning by early adulthood and present in a variety of contexts, as indicated by five (or more) of the following:
    1. Frantic efforts to avoid real or imagined abandonment.
    2. A pattern of unstable and intense interpersonal relationships characterized by alternating between extremes of idealization and devaluation.

3. Identity disturbance: markedly and persistently unstable self-image or sense of self.
4. Impulsivity in at least two areas that are potentially self-damaging (e.g., spending, sex, substance abuse, reckless driving, binge eating).
5. Recurrent suicidal behavior, gestures, or threats, or self-mutilating behavior.
6. Affective instability due to a marked reactivity of mood (e.g., intense episodic dysphoria, irritability, or anxiety usually lasting a few hours and only rarely more than a few days).
7. Chronic feelings of emptiness.
8. Inappropriate, intense anger or difficulty controlling anger (e.g., frequent displays of temper, constant anger, recurrent physical fights).
9. Transient, stress-related paranoid ideation or severe dissociative symptoms.

2. Antisocial Personality Disorder (ASPD)

- **A pervasive pattern of disregard for and violation of the rights of others**, occurring since age 15 years, as indicated by three (or more) of the following:
    1. Failure to conform to social norms with respect to lawful behaviors, as indicated by repeatedly performing acts that are grounds for arrest.
    2. Deceitfulness, as indicated by repeated lying, use of aliases, or conning others for personal profit or pleasure.
    3. Impulsivity or failure to plan ahead.

4. Irritability and aggressiveness, as indicated by repeated physical fights or assaults.
5. Reckless disregard for the safety of self or others.
6. Consistent irresponsibility, as indicated by repeated failure to sustain consistent work behavior or honor financial obligations.
7. Lack of remorse, as indicated by being indifferent to or rationalizing having hurt, mistreated, or stolen from another.

- **The individual is at least age 18 years.**
- **There is evidence of conduct disorder with onset before age 15 years.**
- **The occurrence of antisocial behavior is not exclusively during the course of schizophrenia or bipolar disorder.**

3. Avoidant Personality Disorder (AVPD)

- **A pervasive pattern of social inhibition, feelings of inadequacy, and hypersensitivity to negative evaluation**, beginning by early adulthood and present in a variety of contexts, as indicated by four (or more) of the following:
  1. Avoids occupational activities that involve significant interpersonal contact because of fears of criticism, disapproval, or rejection.
  2. Is unwilling to get involved with people unless certain of being liked.
  3. Shows restraint within intimate relationships because of the fear of being shamed or ridiculed.

4. Is preoccupied with being criticized or rejected in social situations.
5. Is inhibited in new interpersonal situations because of feelings of inadequacy.
6. Views self as socially inept, personally unappealing, or inferior to others.
7. Is unusually reluctant to take personal risks or to engage in any new activities because they may prove embarrassing.

Case Study

Case Study: Jane

Jane is a 28-year-old woman who has struggled with intense and unstable relationships, a fluctuating sense of self, and impulsive behaviors since her teenage years. She often feels empty and fears abandonment, leading her to make frantic efforts to avoid real or imagined separation from others. Jane's mood changes rapidly, and she experiences episodes of intense anger and depression.

Jane's symptoms include:

- **Fear of Abandonment:** Jane goes to great lengths to avoid being abandoned, such as threatening self-harm if her partner talks about leaving.
- **Unstable Relationships:** Her relationships are characterized by extreme ups and downs. She alternates between idealizing her partners and then devaluing them after minor disagreements.

- **Identity Disturbance:** Jane has an unstable self-image. She often feels like she doesn't know who she is or what she wants in life.
- **Impulsivity:** She engages in impulsive behaviors such as binge eating, spending sprees, and unsafe sexual practices.
- **Self-Harm:** Jane has a history of self-mutilation and has made several suicide attempts during periods of intense distress.
- **Mood Instability:** Her mood shifts rapidly from intense happiness to deep depression within hours.
- **Chronic Emptiness:** She frequently feels empty and bored, leading her to engage in risky behaviors to fill the void.
- **Intense Anger:** Jane has difficulty controlling her anger. She often has outbursts of rage that are disproportionate to the situation.
- **Paranoid Ideation:** Under stress, Jane experiences transient paranoid thoughts and dissociative symptoms, feeling detached from reality.

Concerned about her mental health, Jane sought help from a mental health professional. After a thorough evaluation, she was diagnosed with Borderline Personality Disorder (BPD). Her treatment plan included Dialectical Behavior Therapy (DBT), which focuses on teaching skills to manage emotions, improve relationships, and reduce self-destructive behaviors.

DBT helped Jane develop coping strategies to deal with her intense emotions and impulsive behaviors. She learned techniques for emotional regulation, distress tolerance, and interpersonal effectiveness. Over time, Jane began to see improvements in her ability to manage her emotions and maintain more stable relationships.

Jane's case highlights the complexity of Borderline Personality Disorder and the importance of specialized therapeutic approaches like DBT in helping individuals manage their symptoms and improve their quality of life.

Extended Case Study: Antisocial Personality Disorder

Case Study: Tom

Tom is a 35-year-old man who has a long history of criminal behavior, deceitfulness, and lack of regard for the rights of others. He has been arrested multiple times for theft, assault, and drug-related offenses. Tom is known for his charming and manipulative behavior, which he uses to deceive others for his personal gain.

Tom's symptoms include:

- **Criminal Behavior:** Tom frequently engages in activities that are grounds for arrest. He has been involved in theft, burglary, and assault.
- **Deceitfulness:** He often lies, uses aliases, and cons others to obtain money or other benefits.

- **Impulsivity:** Tom acts without considering the consequences, often getting into trouble due to his impulsive actions.
- **Aggressiveness:** He has a history of physical fights and violent outbursts.
- **Recklessness:** He shows a reckless disregard for his own safety and the safety of others, engaging in dangerous activities without concern for potential harm.
- **Irresponsibility:** Tom has difficulty maintaining steady employment and often fails to meet his financial obligations.
- **Lack of Remorse:** He shows no remorse for his actions, rationalizing his behavior and blaming his victims for their misfortune.

Tom's behavior led to a court-ordered psychological evaluation after his latest arrest. The evaluation revealed a pattern of antisocial behavior dating back to his teenage years, consistent with a diagnosis of Antisocial Personality Disorder (ASPD). His treatment plan included psychotherapy aimed at addressing his impulsive behaviors and lack of empathy.

Therapy focused on helping Tom understand the impact of his actions on others and develop a sense of responsibility. Cognitive-behavioral therapy (CBT) techniques were used to address his distorted thinking patterns and promote pro-social behavior. While progress was slow due to the pervasive nature of his disorder, Tom began to make small improvements in his behavior and decision-making.

Tom's case highlights the challenges of treating Antisocial Personality Disorder and the importance of long-term, consistent therapeutic interventions. With persistent effort, individuals with ASPD can make changes that lead to improved functioning and reduced criminal behavior.

Summarized Charts

Neurodevelopmental Disorders

Autism Spectrum Disorder (ASD)

Criteria	Details
Key Symptoms	Persistent deficits in social communication and interaction; restricted, repetitive patterns of behavior, interests, or activities
Duration	Symptoms present from early developmental period
Impairment	Significant impairment in social, occupational, or other important areas of functioning
Exclusions	Not better explained by intellectual disability or global developmental delay
Treatment Options	Behavioral therapy, speech therapy, occupational therapy, educational interventions, medications for co-occurring conditions
Notes	Early diagnosis and intervention are crucial for better outcomes

Attention-Deficit/Hyperactivity Disorder (ADHD)

Criteria	Details
Key Symptoms	Persistent pattern of inattention and/or hyperactivity-impulsivity that interferes with functioning or development
Duration	Symptoms present for at least 6 months
Impairment	Significant impairment in social, academic, or occupational functioning
Exclusions	Not better explained by another mental disorder
Treatment Options	Behavioral therapy, stimulant medications, non-stimulant medications, educational interventions
Notes	Early diagnosis and treatment can significantly improve outcomes

Intellectual Disability

Criteria	Details
Key Symptoms	Deficits in intellectual functioning and adaptive functioning in conceptual, social, and practical domains
Duration	Onset during the developmental period
Impairment	Significant impairment in intellectual and adaptive functioning
Exclusions	Not better explained by another mental disorder
Treatment Options	Special education, behavioral therapy, speech therapy, occupational therapy
Notes	Early intervention and support are crucial

Specific Learning Disorder

Criteria	Details
Key Symptoms	Difficulties learning and using academic skills, significantly below age expectations
Duration	Persistent difficulties for at least 6 months despite targeted interventions
Impairment	Significant impairment in academic functioning
Exclusions	Not better explained by intellectual disabilities, uncorrected visual or auditory acuity, other mental or neurological disorders
Treatment Options	Educational interventions, specialized instruction, accommodations
Notes	Early identification and support are key to academic success

Schizophrenia Spectrum and Other Psychotic Disorders

Schizophrenia

Criteria	Details
Key Symptoms	Delusions, hallucinations, disorganized speech, grossly disorganized or catatonic behavior, negative symptoms
Duration	Continuous signs of disturbance for at least 6 months, including 1 month of active-phase symptoms
Impairment	Significant impairment in social, occupational, or other important areas of functioning
Exclusions	Not attributable to the physiological effects of a substance or another medical condition
Treatment Options	Antipsychotic medications, cognitive-behavioral therapy (CBT), supportive therapy, psychosocial interventions
Notes	Early intervention and comprehensive treatment improve outcomes

Schizoaffective Disorder

Criteria	Details
Key Symptoms	Major mood episode (depressive or manic) concurrent with symptoms of schizophrenia
Duration	Symptoms present for a significant portion of the illness
Impairment	Significant impairment in social, occupational, or other important areas of functioning
Exclusions	Not attributable to the physiological effects of a substance or another medical condition
Treatment Options	Antipsychotic medications, mood stabilizers, psychotherapy, psychosocial interventions
Notes	Integrated treatment for mood and psychotic symptoms is essential

Brief Psychotic Disorder

Criteria	Details
Key Symptoms	Delusions, hallucinations, disorganized speech, grossly disorganized or catatonic behavior
Duration	Symptoms last at least 1 day but less than 1 month
Impairment	Return to premorbid level of functioning after the episode
Exclusions	Not better explained by a mood disorder with psychotic features, schizophrenia, or another psychotic disorder
Treatment Options	Antipsychotic medications, psychotherapy, supportive therapy
Notes	Short duration of symptoms distinguishes this disorder from other psychotic disorders

Delusional Disorder

Criteria	Details
Key Symptoms	Presence of one or more delusions with a duration of 1 month or longer
Duration	Delusions present for at least 1 month
Impairment	Functioning is not markedly impaired, and behavior is not obviously odd or bizarre
Exclusions	Not better explained by schizophrenia, mood disorder with psychotic features, or another psychotic disorder
Treatment Options	Antipsychotic medications, psychotherapy, supportive therapy
Notes	Delusions are the primary symptom, with relatively preserved functioning

Bipolar and Related Disorders

Bipolar I Disorder

Criteria	Details
Key Symptoms	Manic episodes with elevated mood, increased activity, decreased need for sleep; depressive episodes
Duration	Symptoms of mania for at least 1 week; depressive episodes lasting at least 2 weeks
Impairment	Significant impairment in social, occupational, or other important areas of functioning
Exclusions	Not attributable to the physiological effects of a substance or another medical condition
Treatment Options	Mood stabilizers, antipsychotic medications, psychotherapy, lifestyle changes
Notes	Monitoring and managing mood episodes are essential for stability

Bipolar II Disorder

Criteria	Details
Key Symptoms	Hypomanic episodes with elevated mood, increased activity, decreased need for sleep; depressive episodes
Duration	Symptoms of hypomania for at least 4 days; depressive episodes lasting at least 2 weeks
Impairment	Significant impairment in social, occupational, or other important areas of functioning
Exclusions	Not attributable to the physiological effects of a substance or another medical condition
Treatment Options	Mood stabilizers, antipsychotic medications, psychotherapy, lifestyle changes
Notes	Hypomanic episodes are less severe than manic episodes but still require treatment

Cyclothymic Disorder

Criteria	Details
Key Symptoms	Numerous periods of hypomanic symptoms and depressive symptoms that do not meet criteria for a hypomanic episode or a major depressive episode
Duration	Symptoms present for at least 2 years (1 year for children and adolescents)
Impairment	Significant impairment in social, occupational, or other important areas of functioning
Exclusions	Not attributable to the physiological effects of a substance or another medical condition
Treatment Options	Mood stabilizers, psychotherapy, lifestyle changes
Notes	Chronic mood fluctuations require ongoing management

Depressive Disorders

Major Depressive Disorder (MDD)

Criteria	Details
Key Symptoms	Depressed mood, loss of interest or pleasure, significant weight change, insomnia or hypersomnia, fatigue, feelings of worthlessness, diminished ability to think or concentrate, recurrent thoughts of death
Duration	Symptoms present for at least 2 weeks
Impairment	Significant impairment in social, occupational, or other important areas of functioning
Exclusions	Not due to substance use, medication, or another medical condition
Treatment Options	Antidepressant medication, cognitive-behavioral therapy (CBT), psychotherapy, lifestyle changes
Notes	Early intervention and comprehensive treatment improve outcomes

Persistent Depressive Disorder (Dysthymia)

Criteria	Details
Key Symptoms	Depressed mood for most of the day, for more days than not, for at least 2 years (1 year for children and adolescents)
Duration	Symptoms present for at least 2 years (1 year for children and adolescents)
Impairment	Significant impairment in social, occupational, or other important areas of functioning
Exclusions	Not due to substance use, medication, or another medical condition
Treatment Options	Antidepressant medication, cognitive-behavioral therapy (CBT), psychotherapy, lifestyle changes
Notes	Chronic nature of symptoms requires long-term management

Disruptive Mood Dysregulation Disorder

Criteria	Details
Key Symptoms	Severe recurrent temper outbursts that are grossly out of proportion in intensity or duration to the situation
Duration	Symptoms present for at least 12 months, with no period lasting 3 or more consecutive months without all of the symptoms
Impairment	Significant impairment in social, educational, or other important areas of functioning
Exclusions	Not attributable to the physiological effects of a substance or another medical condition
Treatment Options	Psychotherapy, cognitive-behavioral therapy (CBT), medications
Notes	Diagnosis is not made before age 6 or after age 18

Premenstrual Dysphoric Disorder

Criteria	Details
Key Symptoms	Mood swings, irritability or anger, depressed mood, anxiety, decreased interest in usual activities, difficulty concentrating, fatigue, changes in appetite, sleep disturbances, physical symptoms
Duration	Symptoms present in the final week before the onset of menses, start to improve within a few days after the onset of menses, and become minimal or absent in the week postmenses
Impairment	Significant impairment in social, occupational, or other important areas of functioning
Exclusions	Not attributable to the physiological effects of a substance or another medical condition
Treatment Options	Antidepressant medication, cognitive-behavioral therapy (CBT), lifestyle changes, hormonal treatments
Notes	Tracking symptoms through menstrual cycles can aid in diagnosis and treatment

Anxiety Disorders

Generalized Anxiety Disorder (GAD)

Criteria	Details
Key Symptoms	Excessive anxiety and worry, difficulty controlling worry, restlessness, fatigue, difficulty concentrating, irritability, muscle tension, sleep disturbance
Duration	Symptoms present for at least 6 months
Impairment	Significant impairment in social, occupational, or other important areas of functioning
Exclusions	Not attributable to the physiological effects of a substance or another medical condition
Treatment Options	Cognitive-behavioral therapy (CBT), medications (SSRIs), lifestyle changes
Notes	Effective management includes both therapy and medications

Panic Disorder

Criteria	Details
Key Symptoms	Recurrent unexpected panic attacks, persistent concern or worry about additional panic attacks or their consequences, significant maladaptive change in behavior related to the attacks
Duration	Symptoms present for at least 1 month
Impairment	Significant impairment in social, occupational, or other important areas of functioning
Exclusions	Not attributable to the physiological effects of a substance or another medical condition
Treatment Options	Cognitive-behavioral therapy (CBT), medications (SSRIs, benzodiazepines), lifestyle changes
Notes	Understanding and managing triggers can help reduce the frequency of panic attacks

Social Anxiety Disorder (Social Phobia)

Criteria	Details
Key Symptoms	Marked fear or anxiety about one or more social situations in which the individual is exposed to possible scrutiny by others
Duration	Symptoms present for at least 6 months
Impairment	Significant impairment in social, occupational, or other important areas of functioning
Exclusions	Not attributable to the physiological effects of a substance or another medical condition
Treatment Options	Cognitive-behavioral therapy (CBT), medications (SSRIs, beta-blockers), exposure therapy
Notes	Early intervention can help manage symptoms and improve social functioning

Specific Phobia

Criteria	Details
Key Symptoms	Marked fear or anxiety about a specific object or situation, which is actively avoided or endured with intense fear or anxiety
Duration	Symptoms present for at least 6 months
Impairment	Significant impairment in social, occupational, or other important areas of functioning
Exclusions	Not attributable to the physiological effects of a substance or another medical condition
Treatment Options	Cognitive-behavioral therapy (CBT), exposure therapy, medications (SSRIs, benzodiazepines)
Notes	Gradual exposure to the feared object or situation can help reduce fear

Separation Anxiety Disorder

Criteria	Details
Key Symptoms	Developmentally inappropriate and excessive fear or anxiety concerning separation from those to whom the individual is attached
Duration	Symptoms present for at least 4 weeks in children and adolescents, and 6 months or more in adults
Impairment	Significant impairment in social, academic, occupational, or other important areas of functioning
Exclusions	Not attributable to the physiological effects of a substance or another medical condition
Treatment Options	Cognitive-behavioral therapy (CBT), family therapy, medications (SSRIs)
Notes	Early intervention and support from caregivers are crucial

Obsessive-Compulsive and Related Disorders

Obsessive-Compulsive Disorder (OCD)

Criteria	Details
Key Symptoms	Obsessions (recurrent, persistent thoughts) and compulsions (repetitive behaviors) that are time-consuming or cause distress
Duration	Obsessions and compulsions are time-consuming (more than 1 hour per day) or cause distress
Impairment	Significant impairment in social, occupational, or other important areas of functioning
Exclusions	Not attributable to the physiological effects of a substance or another medical condition
Treatment Options	Cognitive-behavioral therapy (CBT), medications (SSRIs), exposure and response prevention (ERP)
Notes	Early intervention and comprehensive treatment improve outcomes

Body Dysmorphic Disorder

Criteria	Details
Key Symptoms	Preoccupation with one or more perceived defects or flaws in physical appearance that are not observable or appear slight to others
Duration	Persistent preoccupation causing significant distress
Impairment	Significant impairment in social, occupational, or other important areas of functioning
Exclusions	Not attributable to the physiological effects of a substance or another medical condition
Treatment Options	Cognitive-behavioral therapy (CBT), medications (SSRIs)
Notes	Recognizing and challenging distorted body image perceptions is crucial

Hoarding Disorder

Criteria	Details
Key Symptoms	Persistent difficulty discarding or parting with possessions, regardless of their actual value
Duration	Persistent difficulty leading to the accumulation of possessions that congest and clutter active living areas
Impairment	Significant impairment in social, occupational, or other important areas of functioning
Exclusions	Not attributable to the physiological effects of a substance or another medical condition
Treatment Options	Cognitive-behavioral therapy (CBT), medications (SSRIs)
Notes	Understanding the emotional attachment to possessions can aid in treatment

Trichotillomania (Hair-Pulling Disorder)

Criteria	Details
Key Symptoms	Recurrent pulling out of one's hair, resulting in hair loss; repeated attempts to decrease or stop hair pulling
Duration	Persistent hair-pulling behavior
Impairment	Significant impairment in social, occupational, or other important areas of functioning
Exclusions	Not attributable to the physiological effects of a substance or another medical condition
Treatment Options	Cognitive-behavioral therapy (CBT), habit reversal training, medications (SSRIs)
Notes	Developing alternative coping mechanisms is essential

Excoriation (Skin-Picking) Disorder

Criteria	Details
Key Symptoms	Recurrent skin-picking resulting in skin lesions; repeated attempts to decrease or stop skin-picking
Duration	Persistent skin-picking behavior
Impairment	Significant impairment in social, occupational, or other important areas of functioning
Exclusions	Not attributable to the physiological effects of a substance or another medical condition
Treatment Options	Cognitive-behavioral therapy (CBT), habit reversal training, medications (SSRIs)
Notes	Addressing underlying stress or anxiety is key to treatment

Trauma and Stressor-Related Disorders

Posttraumatic Stress Disorder (PTSD)

Criteria	Details
Key Symptoms	Exposure to trauma, intrusive memories, avoidance, negative changes in thought and mood, changes in physical and emotional reactions
Duration	Symptoms present for more than 1 month
Impairment	Significant impairment in social, occupational, or other important areas of functioning
Exclusions	Not attributable to the physiological effects of a substance or another medical condition
Treatment Options	Trauma-focused therapy, cognitive-behavioral therapy (CBT), medications (SSRIs), support groups
Notes	Supportive environment and trauma-focused therapy are crucial

Acute Stress Disorder

Criteria	Details
Key Symptoms	Exposure to trauma, intrusive memories, avoidance, negative changes in thought and mood, changes in physical and emotional reactions
Duration	Symptoms last from 3 days to 1 month following trauma exposure
Impairment	Significant impairment in social, occupational, or other important areas of functioning
Exclusions	Not attributable to the physiological effects of a substance or another medical condition
Treatment Options	Trauma-focused therapy, cognitive-behavioral therapy (CBT), medications (SSRIs), support groups
Notes	Early intervention can prevent progression to PTSD

Adjustment Disorders

Criteria	Details
Key Symptoms	Emotional or behavioral symptoms in response to an identifiable stressor(s) occurring within 3 months of the onset of the stressor(s)
Duration	Symptoms persist for no longer than 6 months after the stressor or its consequences have ceased
Impairment	Significant impairment in social, occupational, or other important areas of functioning
Exclusions	Not attributable to the physiological effects of a substance or another medical condition
Treatment Options	Psychotherapy, cognitive-behavioral therapy (CBT), support groups
Notes	Understanding and addressing the stressor is key to treatment

Reactive Attachment Disorder

Criteria	Details
Key Symptoms	Consistent pattern of inhibited, emotionally withdrawn behavior toward adult caregivers, minimal social and emotional responsiveness to others, limited positive affect, episodes of unexplained irritability, sadness, or fearfulness during interactions with adult caregivers
Duration	Symptoms present before age 5
Impairment	Significant impairment in social, occupational, or other important areas of functioning
Exclusions	Not attributable to the physiological effects of a substance or another medical condition
Treatment Options	Psychotherapy, family therapy, play therapy
Notes	Early intervention and a stable caregiving environment are crucial

Disinhibited Social Engagement Disorder

Criteria	Details
Key Symptoms	Pattern of behavior in which a child actively approaches and interacts with unfamiliar adults, overly familiar verbal or physical behavior, diminished or absent checking back with adult caregivers, willingness to go off with an unfamiliar adult
Duration	Symptoms present before age 5
Impairment	Significant impairment in social, occupational, or other important areas of functioning
Exclusions	Not attributable to the physiological effects of a substance or another medical condition
Treatment Options	Psychotherapy, family therapy, play therapy
Notes	Early intervention and a stable caregiving environment are crucial

Dissociative Disorders

Dissociative Identity Disorder (DID)

Criteria	Details
Key Symptoms	Two or more distinct personality states, recurrent gaps in recall of everyday events, significant distress or impairment
Duration	Symptoms present for an extended period, often starting in childhood
Impairment	Significant impairment in social, occupational, or other important areas of functioning
Exclusions	Not attributable to the physiological effects of a substance or another medical condition
Treatment Options	Psychotherapy, cognitive-behavioral therapy (CBT), trauma-focused therapy
Notes	Early intervention and comprehensive treatment improve outcomes

Dissociative Amnesia

Criteria	Details
Key Symptoms	Inability to recall important autobiographical information, usually of a traumatic or stressful nature, that is inconsistent with ordinary forgetting
Duration	Symptoms present for an extended period
Impairment	Significant impairment in social, occupational, or other important areas of functioning
Exclusions	Not attributable to the physiological effects of a substance or another medical condition
Treatment Options	Psychotherapy, cognitive-behavioral therapy (CBT), trauma-focused therapy
Notes	Addressing underlying trauma is crucial for treatment

Depersonalization/Derealization Disorder

Criteria	Details
Key Symptoms	Persistent or recurrent experiences of depersonalization (feeling detached from one's self) and/or derealization (experiences of unreality or detachment from surroundings)
Duration	Persistent or recurrent symptoms
Impairment	Significant impairment in social, occupational, or other important areas of functioning
Exclusions	Not attributable to the physiological effects of a substance or another medical condition
Treatment Options	Psychotherapy, cognitive-behavioral therapy (CBT), medications
Notes	Understanding the nature of dissociation can aid in treatment

Somatic Symptom and Related Disorders

Somatic Symptom Disorder

Criteria	Details
Key Symptoms	One or more somatic symptoms causing distress; excessive thoughts, feelings, or behaviors related to symptoms
Duration	Symptoms persist for more than 6 months
Impairment	Significant impairment in social, occupational, or other important areas of functioning
Exclusions	Not attributable to the physiological effects of a substance or another medical condition
Treatment Options	Cognitive-behavioral therapy (CBT), medications, mindfulness-based stress reduction (MBSR)
Notes	Understanding the psychological component is key to treatment

Illness Anxiety Disorder

Criteria	Details
Key Symptoms	Preoccupation with having or acquiring a serious illness, high level of anxiety about health, excessive health-related behaviors
Duration	Symptoms present for at least 6 months
Impairment	Significant impairment in social, occupational, or other important areas of functioning
Exclusions	Not attributable to the physiological effects of a substance or another medical condition
Treatment Options	Cognitive-behavioral therapy (CBT), medications, mindfulness-based stress reduction (MBSR)
Notes	Reassurance and education about health anxiety are crucial

Conversion Disorder (Functional Neurological Symptom Disorder)

Criteria	Details
Key Symptoms	One or more symptoms of altered voluntary motor or sensory function that are inconsistent with recognized neurological or medical conditions
Duration	Persistent symptoms causing distress
Impairment	Significant impairment in social, occupational, or other important areas of functioning
Exclusions	Not attributable to the physiological effects of a substance or another medical condition
Treatment Options	Cognitive-behavioral therapy (CBT), physical therapy, psychotherapy
Notes	Addressing psychological factors and reinforcing healthy behaviors are crucial

Factitious Disorder

Criteria	Details
Key Symptoms	Falsification of physical or psychological symptoms, or induction of injury or disease, associated with identified deception
Duration	Persistent deceptive behavior
Impairment	Significant impairment in social, occupational, or other important areas of functioning
Exclusions	Not attributable to the physiological effects of a substance or another medical condition
Treatment Options	Psychotherapy, cognitive-behavioral therapy (CBT), addressing underlying psychological needs
Notes	Confronting the deceptive behavior in a nonjudgmental manner is important

Feeding and Eating Disorders

Anorexia Nervosa

Criteria	Details
Key Symptoms	Restriction of energy intake, intense fear of gaining weight, disturbance in self-perceived weight or shape
Duration	Symptoms present for at least 3 months
Impairment	Significant impairment in social, occupational, or other important areas of functioning
Exclusions	Not attributable to the physiological effects of a substance or another medical condition
Treatment Options	Nutritional rehabilitation, cognitive-behavioral therapy (CBT), family-based therapy
Notes	Early intervention and comprehensive treatment improve outcomes

Bulimia Nervosa

Criteria	Details
Key Symptoms	Recurrent episodes of binge eating, followed by inappropriate compensatory behaviors (e.g., vomiting, excessive exercise) to prevent weight gain
Duration	Symptoms present for at least 3 months
Impairment	Significant impairment in social, occupational, or other important areas of functioning
Exclusions	Not attributable to the physiological effects of a substance or another medical condition
Treatment Options	Nutritional counseling, cognitive-behavioral therapy (CBT), medications (SSRIs)
Notes	Addressing both the binge eating and compensatory behaviors is crucial

Binge-Eating Disorder

Criteria	Details
Key Symptoms	Recurrent episodes of binge eating without the use of inappropriate compensatory behaviors
Duration	Symptoms present for at least 3 months
Impairment	Significant impairment in social, occupational, or other important areas of functioning
Exclusions	Not attributable to the physiological effects of a substance or another medical condition
Treatment Options	Nutritional counseling, cognitive-behavioral therapy (CBT), medications (SSRIs)
Notes	Focusing on healthy eating habits and managing triggers for binge eating is essential

Pica

Criteria	Details
Key Symptoms	Persistent eating of non-nutritive, non-food substances
Duration	Symptoms present for at least 1 month
Impairment	Significant impairment in social, occupational, or other important areas of functioning
Exclusions	Not attributable to the physiological effects of a substance or another medical condition
Treatment Options	Nutritional counseling, behavioral therapy
Notes	Addressing underlying nutritional deficiencies and behavioral aspects is key

Rumination Disorder

Criteria	Details
Key Symptoms	Repeated regurgitation of food, which may be re-chewed, re-swallowed, or spit out
Duration	Symptoms present for at least 1 month
Impairment	Significant impairment in social, occupational, or other important areas of functioning
Exclusions	Not attributable to the physiological effects of a substance or another medical condition
Treatment Options	Behavioral therapy, family therapy
Notes	Early intervention and addressing behavioral patterns are crucial

Sleep-Wake Disorders

Insomnia Disorder

Criteria	Details
Key Symptoms	Difficulty initiating or maintaining sleep, early-morning awakening, distress or impairment in daily functioning
Duration	Symptoms occur at least 3 nights per week for at least 3 months
Impairment	Significant impairment in social, occupational, educational, academic, or other areas of functioning
Exclusions	Not attributable to the physiological effects of a substance or another medical condition
Treatment Options	Cognitive-behavioral therapy for insomnia (CBT-I), medications, sleep hygiene education
Notes	Good sleep hygiene practices are crucial for effective management

Hypersomnolence Disorder

Criteria	Details
Key Symptoms	Excessive sleepiness despite a main sleep period lasting at least 7 hours, difficulty being fully awake after abrupt awakening
Duration	Symptoms occur at least three times per week for at least 3 months
Impairment	Significant impairment in social, occupational, or other important areas of functioning
Exclusions	Not attributable to the physiological effects of a substance or another medical condition
Treatment Options	Stimulant medications, cognitive-behavioral therapy (CBT), lifestyle changes
Notes	Understanding and managing sleep patterns is essential

Narcolepsy

Criteria	Details
Key Symptoms	Recurrent periods of an irrepressible need to sleep, lapsing into sleep, or napping occurring within the same day
Duration	Symptoms occur at least three times per week for at least 3 months
Impairment	Significant impairment in social, occupational, or other important areas of functioning
Exclusions	Not attributable to the physiological effects of a substance or another medical condition
Treatment Options	Stimulant medications, lifestyle modifications, cognitive-behavioral therapy (CBT)
Notes	Managing sleep attacks and ensuring safety is crucial

Obstructive Sleep Apnea Hypopnea

Criteria	Details
Key Symptoms	Recurrent episodes of upper airway obstruction during sleep, resulting in disrupted sleep and excessive daytime sleepiness
Duration	Persistent symptoms occurring regularly
Impairment	Significant impairment in social, occupational, or other important areas of functioning
Exclusions	Not attributable to the physiological effects of a substance or another medical condition
Treatment Options	Continuous positive airway pressure (CPAP), lifestyle changes, weight management
Notes	Early diagnosis and treatment can prevent complications

Circadian Rhythm Sleep-Wake Disorders

Criteria	Details
Key Symptoms	Persistent or recurrent pattern of sleep disruption due to alteration of the circadian system or misalignment between endogenous circadian rhythm and the sleep-wake schedule required by an individual's physical environment or social or professional schedule
Duration	Persistent symptoms causing distress
Impairment	Significant impairment in social, occupational, or other important areas of functioning
Exclusions	Not attributable to the physiological effects of a substance or another medical condition
Treatment Options	Bright light therapy, chronotherapy, melatonin supplements
Notes	Aligning sleep-wake schedule with circadian rhythm is essential

Parasomnias

Criteria	Details
Key Symptoms	Abnormal behavioral, experiential, or physiological events occurring in association with sleep, specific sleep stages, or sleep-wake transitions
Duration	Persistent symptoms causing distress
Impairment	Significant impairment in social, occupational, or other important areas of functioning
Exclusions	Not attributable to the physiological effects of a substance or another medical condition
Treatment Options	Safety measures, cognitive-behavioral therapy (CBT), medications
Notes	Understanding the type of parasomnia is crucial for treatment

Sexual Dysfunctions

Erectile Disorder

Criteria	Details
Key Symptoms	Difficulty obtaining or maintaining an erection, decreased erectile rigidity, significant distress
Duration	Symptoms persist for at least 6 months
Impairment	Significant impairment in social, occupational, or other important areas of functioning
Exclusions	Not attributable to the physiological effects of a substance or another medical condition
Treatment Options	Medications (PDE5 inhibitors), psychotherapy, lifestyle changes
Notes	Address both psychological and physical aspects of the disorder

Female Sexual Interest/Arousal Disorder

Criteria	Details
Key Symptoms	Lack of, or significantly reduced, sexual interest/arousal
Duration	Symptoms present for at least 6 months
Impairment	Significant impairment in social, occupational, or other important areas of functioning
Exclusions	Not attributable to the physiological effects of a substance or another medical condition
Treatment Options	Psychotherapy, hormonal therapy, lifestyle changes
Notes	Understanding underlying psychological or medical factors is crucial

Genito-Pelvic Pain/Penetration Disorder

Criteria	Details
Key Symptoms	Difficulty with vaginal penetration during intercourse, vulvovaginal or pelvic pain, fear or anxiety about pain, tensing or tightening of pelvic floor muscles
Duration	Symptoms present for at least 6 months
Impairment	Significant impairment in social, occupational, or other important areas of functioning
Exclusions	Not attributable to the physiological effects of a substance or another medical condition
Treatment Options	Psychotherapy, physical therapy, relaxation techniques
Notes	Multidisciplinary approach can be effective

Male Hypoactive Sexual Desire Disorder

Criteria	Details
Key Symptoms	Persistently or recurrently deficient (or absent) sexual/erotic thoughts or fantasies and desire for sexual activity
Duration	Symptoms present for at least 6 months
Impairment	Significant impairment in social, occupational, or other important areas of functioning
Exclusions	Not attributable to the physiological effects of a substance or another medical condition
Treatment Options	Psychotherapy, hormonal therapy, lifestyle changes
Notes	Understanding underlying psychological or medical factors is crucial

Premature (Early) Ejaculation

Criteria	Details
Key Symptoms	Persistent or recurrent pattern of ejaculation occurring during partnered sexual activity within approximately 1 minute following vaginal penetration and before the individual wishes it
Duration	Symptoms present for at least 6 months
Impairment	Significant impairment in social, occupational, or other important areas of functioning
Exclusions	Not attributable to the physiological effects of a substance or another medical condition
Treatment Options	Psychotherapy, behavioral techniques, medications (SSRIs)
Notes	Addressing both psychological and physical aspects of the disorder is crucial

Oppositional Defiant Disorder (ODD)

Criteria	Details
Key Symptoms	Angry/irritable mood, argumentative/defiant behavior, vindictiveness
Duration	Pattern of behavior lasting at least 6 months
Impairment	Significant impairment in social, educational, occupational, or other areas of functioning
Exclusions	Not occurring exclusively during the course of another mental disorder
Treatment Options	Parent management training, cognitive-behavioral therapy (CBT), family therapy
Notes	Consistency and structure are key in managing symptoms

Disruptive, Impulse-Control, and Conduct Disorders

Conduct Disorder

Criteria	Details
Key Symptoms	Repetitive and persistent pattern of behavior that violates the basic rights of others or major age-appropriate societal norms or rules
Duration	Persistent pattern of behavior lasting at least 12 months
Impairment	Significant impairment in social, educational, or other important areas of functioning
Exclusions	Not occurring exclusively during the course of another mental disorder
Treatment Options	Parent management training, cognitive-behavioral therapy (CBT), family therapy, multisystemic therapy
Notes	Early intervention and consistent discipline are crucial

Intermittent Explosive Disorder

Criteria	Details
Key Symptoms	Recurrent behavioral outbursts representing a failure to control aggressive impulses, manifested by verbal or physical aggression
Duration	Aggressive outbursts are grossly out of proportion to the provocation
Impairment	Significant impairment in social, occupational, or other important areas of functioning
Exclusions	Not attributable to the physiological effects of a substance or another medical condition
Treatment Options	Cognitive-behavioral therapy (CBT), medications (SSRIs, mood stabilizers)
Notes	Managing triggers and developing coping strategies are crucial

Antisocial Personality Disorder

Criteria	Details
Key Symptoms	Disregard for and violation of the rights of others, deceitfulness, impulsivity, irritability, aggression, reckless disregard for safety, consistent irresponsibility, lack of remorse
Duration	Persistent pattern of behavior occurring since age 15
Impairment	Significant impairment in social, occupational, or other important areas of functioning
Exclusions	Not attributable to the physiological effects of a substance or another medical condition
Treatment Options	Psychotherapy, cognitive-behavioral therapy (CBT), medications (SSRIs)
Notes	Early intervention and consistent structure are crucial

Pyromania

Criteria	Details
Key Symptoms	Recurrent failure to resist impulses to steal objects not needed for personal use or monetary value, tension before the theft, pleasure or relief at the time of committing the theft
Duration	Persistent stealing behavior
Impairment	Significant impairment in social, occupational, or other important areas of functioning
Exclusions	Not attributable to the physiological effects of a substance or another medical condition
Treatment Options	Cognitive-behavioral therapy (CBT), medications (SSRIs)
Notes	Addressing underlying psychological issues is crucial

Substance-Related and Addictive Disorders

Alcohol Use Disorder

Criteria	Details
Key Symptoms	Problematic pattern of alcohol use leading to impairment or distress, withdrawal symptoms, tolerance
Duration	Symptoms occurring within a 12-month period
Impairment	Significant impairment in social, occupational, or other important areas of functioning
Exclusions	Not attributable to the physiological effects of a substance or another medical condition
Treatment Options	Detoxification, cognitive-behavioral therapy (CBT), motivational interviewing, support groups
Notes	Comprehensive treatment approach yields the best results

Tobacco Use Disorder

Criteria	Details
Key Symptoms	Problematic pattern of tobacco use leading to impairment or distress, withdrawal symptoms, tolerance
Duration	Symptoms occurring within a 12-month period
Impairment	Significant impairment in social, occupational, or other important areas of functioning
Exclusions	Not attributable to the physiological effects of a substance or another medical condition
Treatment Options	Behavioral therapy, nicotine replacement therapy, medications (bupropion, varenicline)
Notes	Support groups and behavioral interventions can enhance success rates

Cannabis Use Disorder

Criteria	Details
Key Symptoms	Problematic pattern of cannabis use leading to impairment or distress, withdrawal symptoms, tolerance
Duration	Symptoms occurring within a 12-month period
Impairment	Significant impairment in social, occupational, or other important areas of functioning
Exclusions	Not attributable to the physiological effects of a substance or another medical condition
Treatment Options	Cognitive-behavioral therapy (CBT), motivational interviewing, support groups
Notes	Comprehensive treatment approach yields the best results

Stimulant Use Disorder

Criteria	Details
Key Symptoms	Problematic pattern of stimulant use leading to impairment or distress, withdrawal symptoms, tolerance
Duration	Symptoms occurring within a 12-month period
Impairment	Significant impairment in social, occupational, or other important areas of functioning
Exclusions	Not attributable to the physiological effects of a substance or another medical condition
Treatment Options	Detoxification, cognitive-behavioral therapy (CBT), motivational interviewing, support groups
Notes	Comprehensive treatment approach yields the best results

Opioid Use Disorder

Criteria	Details
Key Symptoms	Problematic pattern of opioid use leading to impairment or distress, withdrawal symptoms, tolerance
Duration	Symptoms occurring within a 12-month period
Impairment	Significant impairment in social, occupational, or other important areas of functioning
Exclusions	Not attributable to the physiological effects of a substance or another medical condition
Treatment Options	Detoxification, medication-assisted treatment (MAT), cognitive-behavioral therapy (CBT), support groups
Notes	Comprehensive treatment approach yields the best results

Gambling Disorder

Criteria	Details
Key Symptoms	Persistent and recurrent problematic gambling behavior leading to impairment or distress
Duration	Symptoms present for at least 12 months
Impairment	Significant impairment in social, occupational, or other important areas of functioning
Exclusions	Not attributable to the physiological effects of a substance or another medical condition
Treatment Options	Cognitive-behavioral therapy (CBT), support groups, medications (SSRIs)
Notes	Understanding and addressing triggers is crucial

171

Neurocognitive Disorders

Major Neurocognitive Disorder (NCD)

Criteria	Details
Key Symptoms	Significant cognitive decline in one or more cognitive domains, interferes with independence in daily activities
Duration	Significant cognitive decline documented by testing, present for an extended period
Impairment	Interferes with independence in everyday activities
Exclusions	Not occurring exclusively in the context of delirium
Treatment Options	Medications, cognitive rehabilitation, psychotherapy, support groups
Notes	Multifaceted treatment approach enhances quality of life

Mild Neurocognitive Disorder

Criteria	Details
Key Symptoms	Modest cognitive decline in one or more cognitive domains, does not interfere with independence in daily activities
Duration	Modest cognitive decline documented by testing, present for an extended period
Impairment	Does not interfere with independence in everyday activities
Exclusions	Not occurring exclusively in the context of delirium
Treatment Options	Cognitive rehabilitation, lifestyle modifications, support groups
Notes	Early intervention can help slow progression to major NCD

Alzheimer's Disease

Criteria	Details
Key Symptoms	Memory impairment, cognitive decline in at least one other cognitive domain, gradual onset and continuing decline
Duration	Progressive cognitive decline present for an extended period
Impairment	Significant impairment in social, occupational, or other important areas of functioning
Exclusions	Not occurring exclusively in the context of delirium
Treatment Options	Medications (cholinesterase inhibitors, memantine), cognitive rehabilitation, support groups
Notes	Early diagnosis and intervention are crucial for managing symptoms

Vascular Neurocognitive Disorder

Criteria	Details
Key Symptoms	Cognitive decline related to cerebrovascular disease, stepwise progression of symptoms
Duration	Progressive cognitive decline present for an extended period
Impairment	Significant impairment in social, occupational, or other important areas of functioning
Exclusions	Not occurring exclusively in the context of delirium
Treatment Options	Managing cardiovascular risk factors, cognitive rehabilitation, support groups
Notes	Controlling underlying vascular conditions is crucial

Frontotemporal Neurocognitive Disorder

Criteria	Details
Key Symptoms	Prominent changes in personality, behavior, and language
Duration	Progressive cognitive decline present for an extended period
Impairment	Significant impairment in social, occupational, or other important areas of functioning
Exclusions	Not occurring exclusively in the context of delirium
Treatment Options	Medications, cognitive rehabilitation, behavioral interventions, support groups
Notes	Early diagnosis and intervention are crucial for managing symptoms

Lewy Body Dementia

Criteria	Details
Key Symptoms	Fluctuating cognition, recurrent visual hallucinations, motor symptoms similar to Parkinson's disease
Duration	Progressive cognitive decline present for an extended period
Impairment	Significant impairment in social, occupational, or other important areas of functioning
Exclusions	Not occurring exclusively in the context of delirium
Treatment Options	Medications, cognitive rehabilitation, behavioral interventions, support groups
Notes	Sensitivity to antipsychotic medications is common

Traumatic Brain Injury (TBI)

Criteria	Details
Key Symptoms	Cognitive impairments resulting from a head injury, memory loss, attention deficits, impaired executive function
Duration	Cognitive decline present for an extended period
Impairment	Significant impairment in social, occupational, or other important areas of functioning
Exclusions	Not occurring exclusively in the context of delirium
Treatment Options	Cognitive rehabilitation, physical therapy, occupational therapy, support groups
Notes	Early intervention and comprehensive treatment improve outcomes

Substance/Medication-Induced Neurocognitive Disorder

Criteria	Details
Key Symptoms	Cognitive impairments related to substance use or medication
Duration	Cognitive decline present for an extended period
Impairment	Significant impairment in social, occupational, or other important areas of functioning
Exclusions	Not occurring exclusively in the context of delirium
Treatment Options	Substance cessation, cognitive rehabilitation, support groups
Notes	Addressing substance use is crucial for managing symptoms

HIV Infection Neurocognitive Disorder

Criteria	Details
Key Symptoms	Cognitive impairments related to HIV infection
Duration	Cognitive decline present for an extended period
Impairment	Significant impairment in social, occupational, or other important areas of functioning
Exclusions	Not occurring exclusively in the context of delirium
Treatment Options	Antiretroviral therapy (ART), cognitive rehabilitation, support groups
Notes	Managing HIV infection is crucial for cognitive health

Prion Disease

Criteria	Details
Key Symptoms	Rapidly progressive cognitive decline, motor abnormalities
Duration	Rapid progression of symptoms
Impairment	Significant impairment in social, occupational, or other important areas of functioning
Exclusions	Not occurring exclusively in the context of delirium
Treatment Options	Supportive care, palliative care
Notes	Rapid progression necessitates early intervention

Parkinson's Disease

Criteria	Details
Key Symptoms	Motor symptoms (tremor, rigidity, bradykinesia), cognitive decline
Duration	Progressive cognitive decline present for an extended period
Impairment	Significant impairment in social, occupational, or other important areas of functioning
Exclusions	Not occurring exclusively in the context of delirium
Treatment Options	Medications (levodopa), cognitive rehabilitation, physical therapy, support groups
Notes	Managing motor and cognitive symptoms is crucial

Huntington's Disease

Criteria	Details
Key Symptoms	Motor abnormalities (chorea), cognitive decline, psychiatric symptoms
Duration	Progressive cognitive decline present for an extended period
Impairment	Significant impairment in social, occupational, or other important areas of functioning
Exclusions	Not occurring exclusively in the context of delirium
Treatment Options	Medications, cognitive rehabilitation, physical therapy, support groups
Notes	Genetic counseling and early intervention are crucial

Personality Disorders

Borderline Personality Disorder (BPD)

Criteria	Details
Key Symptoms	Instability in interpersonal relationships, self-image, and affects, marked impulsivity
Duration	Symptoms present from early adulthood, pervasive and chronic
Impairment	Significant impairment in social, occupational, or other important areas of functioning
Exclusions	Not attributable to the physiological effects of a substance or another medical condition
Treatment Options	Dialectical behavior therapy (DBT), cognitive-behavioral therapy (CBT), medications for co-occurring conditions
Notes	Specialized therapeutic approaches like DBT are effective

Antisocial Personality Disorder

Criteria	Details
Key Symptoms	Disregard for and violation of the rights of others, deceitfulness, impulsivity, irritability, aggression, reckless disregard for safety, consistent irresponsibility, lack of remorse
Duration	Persistent pattern of behavior occurring since age 15
Impairment	Significant impairment in social, occupational, or other important areas of functioning
Exclusions	Not attributable to the physiological effects of a substance or another medical condition
Treatment Options	Psychotherapy, cognitive-behavioral therapy (CBT), medications (SSRIs)
Notes	Early intervention and consistent structure are crucial

Narcissistic Personality Disorder

Criteria	Details
Key Symptoms	Grandiosity, need for admiration, lack of empathy
Duration	Persistent pattern of behavior
Impairment	Significant impairment in social, occupational, or other important areas of functioning
Exclusions	Not attributable to the physiological effects of a substance or another medical condition
Treatment Options	Psychotherapy, cognitive-behavioral therapy (CBT)
Notes	Building empathy and addressing grandiosity are key to treatment

Histrionic Personality Disorder

Criteria	Details
Key Symptoms	Excessive emotionality, attention-seeking behavior
Duration	Persistent pattern of behavior
Impairment	Significant impairment in social, occupational, or other important areas of functioning
Exclusions	Not attributable to the physiological effects of a substance or another medical condition
Treatment Options	Psychotherapy, cognitive-behavioral therapy (CBT)
Notes	Understanding underlying emotional needs is crucial

Avoidant Personality Disorder

Criteria	Details
Key Symptoms	Social inhibition, feelings of inadequacy, hypersensitivity to negative evaluation
Duration	Persistent pattern of behavior
Impairment	Significant impairment in social, occupational, or other important areas of functioning
Exclusions	Not attributable to the physiological effects of a substance or another medical condition
Treatment Options	Psychotherapy, cognitive-behavioral therapy (CBT)
Notes	Building self-esteem and social skills is key to treatment

Dependent Personality Disorder

Criteria	Details
Key Symptoms	Excessive need to be taken care of, submissive and clinging behavior, fears of separation
Duration	Persistent pattern of behavior
Impairment	Significant impairment in social, occupational, or other important areas of functioning
Exclusions	Not attributable to the physiological effects of a substance or another medical condition
Treatment Options	Psychotherapy, cognitive-behavioral therapy (CBT)
Notes	Encouraging independence and self-reliance is crucial

Obsessive-Compulsive Personality Disorder

Criteria	Details
Key Symptoms	Preoccupation with orderliness, perfectionism, and control
Duration	Persistent pattern of behavior
Impairment	Significant impairment in social, occupational, or other important areas of functioning
Exclusions	Not attributable to the physiological effects of a substance or another medical condition
Treatment Options	Psychotherapy, cognitive-behavioral therapy (CBT)
Notes	Addressing perfectionism and need for control is key to treatment

Paranoid Personality Disorder

Criteria	Details
Key Symptoms	Pervasive distrust and suspiciousness of others
Duration	Persistent pattern of behavior
Impairment	Significant impairment in social, occupational, or other important areas of functioning
Exclusions	Not attributable to the physiological effects of a substance or another medical condition
Treatment Options	Psychotherapy, cognitive-behavioral therapy (CBT)
Notes	Building trust and addressing paranoia is crucial

Schizoid Personality Disorder

Criteria	Details
Key Symptoms	Detachment from social relationships, restricted range of emotional expression
Duration	Persistent pattern of behavior
Impairment	Significant impairment in social, occupational, or other important areas of functioning
Exclusions	Not attributable to the physiological effects of a substance or another medical condition
Treatment Options	Psychotherapy, cognitive-behavioral therapy (CBT)
Notes	Developing social skills and emotional expression is key

Schizotypal Personality Disorder

Criteria	Details
Key Symptoms	Acute discomfort in close relationships, cognitive or perceptual distortions, eccentricities of behavior
Duration	Persistent pattern of behavior
Impairment	Significant impairment in social, occupational, or other important areas of functioning
Exclusions	Not attributable to the physiological effects of a substance or another medical condition
Treatment Options	Psychotherapy, cognitive-behavioral therapy (CBT), medications
Notes	Addressing cognitive distortions and social skills is crucial

Part III:

Study Aids and Practice

Mnemonics for DSM-5-TR Disorders

Mnemonics are memory aids that help simplify and remember complex information. They are particularly useful in studying mental health disorders where numerous criteria need to be recalled. Here are mnemonics for a wide range of DSM-5-TR disorders along with explanations on how to use them effectively.

Major Depressive Disorder (MDD)

Mnemonic: SIG E CAPS

- **S**leep disturbances: Insomnia or hypersomnia.
- **I**nterest (loss of): Markedly diminished interest or pleasure in almost all activities.
- **G**uilt or feelings of worthlessness: Excessive or inappropriate guilt.
- **E**nergy (lack of): Fatigue or loss of energy nearly every day.
- **C**oncentration difficulties: Diminished ability to think or concentrate.
- **A**ppetite changes: Significant weight loss or gain, or decrease/increase in appetite.
- **P**sychomotor agitation or retardation: Observable by others, not merely subjective feelings.
- **S**uicidal thoughts: Recurrent thoughts of death, suicidal ideation, or a suicide attempt.

How to Use: The mnemonic "SIG E CAPS" is useful for recalling the core symptoms of Major Depressive Disorder. When diagnosing MDD, ensure that at least five of these symptoms are present for a minimum of two weeks, with at least one symptom being either depressed mood or loss of interest/pleasure.

Bipolar Disorder

Mnemonic: DIG FAST (for Manic Episode)

- **D**istractibility: Easily distracted, unable to focus.
- **I**ndiscretion: Engaging in activities with a high potential for painful consequences (e.g., buying sprees, sexual indiscretions).
- **G**randiosity: Inflated self-esteem or grandiosity.
- **F**light of ideas: Racing thoughts.
- **A**ctivity increase: Increase in goal-directed activities (social, work, school, or sexual).
- **S**leep deficit: Decreased need for sleep (feeling rested after only a few hours of sleep).
- **T**alkativeness: More talkative than usual or pressure to keep talking.

How to Use: "DIG FAST" helps in identifying the symptoms of a manic episode in Bipolar I Disorder. Use this mnemonic to check if the patient exhibits at least three of these symptoms (four if the mood is only irritable) for at least one week.

Generalized Anxiety Disorder (GAD)

Mnemonic: WATCHERS

- **W**orry: Excessive anxiety and worry occurring more days than not.
- **A**nxiety: Excessive, difficult to control.
- **T**ension in muscles: Muscle tension.
- **C**oncentration difficulty: Difficulty concentrating or mind going blank.
- **H**yperarousal (irritability): Irritability.
- **E**nergy loss: Fatigue.
- **R**estlessness: Restlessness or feeling keyed up or on edge.
- **S**leep disturbance: Difficulty falling or staying asleep, or restless, unsatisfying sleep.

How to Use: "WATCHERS" is effective for diagnosing GAD. Check if the patient has excessive worry and at least three of the associated symptoms for at least six months.

Obsessive-Compulsive Disorder (OCD)

Mnemonic: SOAP

- **S**ymmetry obsession: Need for symmetry, exactness, or a specific order.
- **O**rdering compulsions: Arranging items in a specific way.
- **A**ggressive thoughts: Intrusive, distressing thoughts about harming oneself or others.
- **P**urity obsession: Preoccupation with cleanliness or contamination fears.

How to Use: Use "SOAP" to remember common themes in OCD. Evaluate if the patient has obsessions (e.g., thoughts about symmetry, aggression) and/or compulsions (e.g., ordering, cleaning) that are time-consuming and cause significant distress.

Posttraumatic Stress Disorder (PTSD)

Mnemonic: TRAUMA

- **T**rauma: Exposure to actual or threatened death, serious injury, or sexual violence.
- **R**e-experiencing: Intrusive memories, flashbacks, or nightmares.
- **A**voidance: Avoidance of stimuli associated with the trauma.
- **U**nable to function: Significant impairment in social, occupational, or other important areas of functioning.
- **M**onth: Symptoms last more than one month.
- **A**rousal: Increased arousal and reactivity (e.g., hypervigilance, exaggerated startle response).

How to Use: "TRAUMA" helps recall the diagnostic criteria for PTSD. Confirm that the patient has been exposed to trauma and experiences re-experiencing symptoms, avoidance, negative alterations in cognition and mood, and arousal symptoms for more than one month.

Attention-Deficit/Hyperactivity Disorder (ADHD)

Mnemonics: MOAT and RUNS FAST

MOAT (for Inattentive Type)

- **M**istakes: Frequent careless mistakes in schoolwork or other activities.
- **O**rganization: Difficulty organizing tasks and activities.
- **A**ttention: Difficulty sustaining attention in tasks or play activities.
- **T**asks: Avoids or is reluctant to engage in tasks requiring sustained mental effort.

RUNS FAST (for Hyperactive-Impulsive Type)

- **R**estlessness: Fidgets with hands or feet or squirms in seat.
- **U**nable to stay seated: Leaves seat in situations when remaining seated is expected.
- **N**oisy: Runs about or climbs excessively in situations where it is inappropriate.
- **S**peaks excessively: Talks excessively.
- **F**idgets: Often fidgets or taps hands or feet.
- **A**nswers out of turn: Blurts out answers before questions have been completed.
- **S**tays on the go: Often "on the go" or acts as if "driven by a motor."
- **T**rouble waiting: Difficulty waiting for their turn.

How to Use: Use "MOAT" to assess inattentive symptoms and "RUNS FAST" to assess hyperactive-impulsive symptoms in ADHD. Check if the patient exhibits six or more symptoms from either category for at least six months.

Panic Disorder

Mnemonic: STUDENTS Fear the 3Cs

- **S**udden onset.
- **T**achycardia (rapid heartbeat).
- **U**ncontrollable shaking or trembling.
- **D**izziness or feeling faint.
- **E**xtreme fear of losing control or "going crazy."
- **N**ausea or abdominal distress.
- **T**ightness in the chest.
- **S**weating.
- **3Cs:** Chills, Choking sensation, Chest pain.

How to Use: "STUDENTS Fear the 3Cs" helps recall the symptoms of a panic attack. Confirm if the patient experiences recurrent unexpected panic attacks and persistent concern or behavior changes related to the attacks for at least one month.

Social Anxiety Disorder

Mnemonic: SCARED

- **S**ocial situations provoke fear.
- **C**riticism or negative evaluation feared.

- Avoidance of social situations.
- Recognizes fear as excessive.
- Exposure causes anxiety.
- Disabling: Impairs daily functioning.

How to Use: "SCARED" aids in diagnosing Social Anxiety Disorder. Assess if the patient consistently fears and avoids social situations, recognizes the fear as excessive, and experiences significant impairment in daily functioning.

Specific Phobia

Mnemonic: FEARED

- Fear of specific objects or situations.
- Exposure causes immediate anxiety response.
- Avoidance behavior or endured with intense fear.
- Recognizes fear as excessive or unreasonable.
- Experience significant distress or impairment in functioning.
- Duration of at least 6 months.

How to Use: "FEARED" helps in identifying Specific Phobia. Check if the patient has a persistent, excessive fear of specific objects or situations, leading to significant distress or impairment for at least six months.

Anorexia Nervosa

Mnemonic: WEIGHT

- **W**eight loss or failure to gain weight during growth.
- **E**ngages in persistent behavior to prevent weight gain.
- **I**ntense fear of gaining weight or becoming fat.
- **G**ross distortion of body image.
- **H**air loss or thinning.
- **T**iredness or fatigue.

How to Use: "WEIGHT" helps recall key symptoms of Anorexia Nervosa. Assess if the patient has significant weight loss, engages in behaviors to prevent weight gain, and has a distorted body image with an intense fear of gaining weight.

Bulimia Nervosa

Mnemonic: BULIMIA

- **B**inge eating: Recurrent episodes.
- **U**ncontrolled eating during binges.
- **L**axatives, diuretics, or other methods to prevent weight gain.
- **I**nterest in body shape and weight.
- **M**inimum of once a week for 3 months.
- **I**mage of body overly influenced by body shape and weight.
- **A**voidance of weight gain by vomiting, excessive exercise, etc.

How to Use: "BULIMIA" assists in diagnosing Bulimia Nervosa. Confirm if the patient has recurrent binge-eating episodes with a lack of control and engages in compensatory behaviors at least once a week for three months.

Binge-Eating Disorder

Mnemonic: BINGE

- **B**inge eating: Recurrent episodes.
- **I**ndividual feels a lack of control during binges.
- **N**ot regularly using compensatory behaviors (like purging).
- **G**uilt or distress about binge eating.
- **E**pisodes occur at least once a week for 3 months.

How to Use: "BINGE" aids in diagnosing Binge-Eating Disorder. Check if the patient has recurrent binge-eating episodes without regular use of compensatory behaviors and experiences distress about binge eating.

Oppositional Defiant Disorder (ODD)

Mnemonic: ARGUE

- **A**rgumentative with authority figures.
- **R**esentful or angry.
- **G**rudges or vindictiveness.
- **U**pset easily by others.
- **E**veryday defiant behavior.

How to Use: "ARGUE" helps identify symptoms of ODD. Confirm if the patient frequently argues with authority figures, is easily upset, and exhibits vindictive behavior for at least six months.

Conduct Disorder

Mnemonic: TRAP

- **T**hreats to people or animals.
- **R**ule violations (serious).
- **A**ggression towards people or animals.
- **P**roperty destruction.

How to Use: "TRAP" aids in identifying Conduct Disorder. Assess if the patient shows aggression towards people or animals, serious rule violations, and property destruction for at least 12 months.

Borderline Personality Disorder (BPD)

Mnemonic: I DESPAIRR

- **I**dentity disturbance.
- **D**isordered and unstable relationships.
- **E**mptiness feelings.
- **S**uicidal or self-harming behaviors.
- **P**aranoia or dissociation under stress.
- **A**bandonment fears.
- **I**mpulsivity in at least two areas.
- **R**age that is inappropriate and intense.

- **R**apidly changing mood (affective instability).

How to Use: "I DESPAIRR" helps recall the criteria for BPD. Confirm if the patient exhibits a pervasive pattern of instability in relationships, self-image, and affect, along with marked impulsivity beginning by early adulthood.

Diagnostic Flowcharts

Diagnostic flowcharts are visual aids that simplify the diagnostic process, helping to distinguish between similar disorders.

They provide a step-by-step approach to diagnosing mental health conditions based on the DSM-5-TR criteria. Below are diagnostic flowcharts for some major disorder categories.

Anxiety Disorders Diagnostic Flowchart

Step 1: Presence of Excessive Worry?

- **Yes:** Go to Step 2.
- **No:** Consider other disorders.

Step 2: Duration of Worry?

- **More than 6 months:** Generalized Anxiety Disorder (GAD)
- **Less than 6 months:** Consider Adjustment Disorder with Anxiety

Step 3: Specific Situations or Objects?

- **Yes:** Evaluate for Specific Phobia or Social Anxiety Disorder (SAD)
- **No:** Go to Step 4.

Step 4: Panic Attacks?

- **Yes:** Consider Panic Disorder
- **No:** Go to Step 5.

Step 5: Fear of Embarrassment or Negative Evaluation?

- **Yes:** Social Anxiety Disorder (SAD)
- **No:** Consider Generalized Anxiety Disorder (GAD) or Specific Phobia

Mood Disorders Diagnostic Flowchart

Step 1: Presence of Depressive Symptoms?

- **Yes:** Go to Step 2.
- **No:** Go to Step 6.

Step 2: Duration of Symptoms?

- **More than 2 weeks:** Major Depressive Disorder (MDD)
- **More than 2 years:** Persistent Depressive Disorder (Dysthymia)
- **Less than 2 weeks:** Consider Adjustment Disorder with Depressed Mood

Step 3: Presence of Manic Symptoms?

- **Yes:** Go to Step 4.
- **No:** Confirm Major Depressive Disorder (MDD) or Persistent Depressive Disorder

Step 4: Severity and Duration of Manic Symptoms?

- **Severe, lasting at least 1 week:** Bipolar I Disorder
- **Hypomanic, lasting at least 4 days:** Bipolar II Disorder

Step 5: Presence of Hypomanic and Depressive Symptoms for at least 2 years?

- **Yes:** Cyclothymic Disorder
- **No:** Re-evaluate symptoms and consider differential diagnoses.

Obsessive-Compulsive and Related Disorders Diagnostic Flowchart

Step 1: Presence of Obsessions and/or Compulsions?

- **Yes:** Go to Step 2.
- **No:** Consider other disorders.

Step 2: Time Consuming or Cause Significant Distress?

- **Yes:** Obsessive-Compulsive Disorder (OCD)
- **No:** Consider subclinical OCD traits or other anxiety disorders.

Step 3: Obsessions Related to Body Image?

- **Yes:** Body Dysmorphic Disorder (BDD)
- **No:** Go to Step 4.

Step 4: Compulsions Involving Hair Pulling or Skin Picking?

- **Hair Pulling:** Trichotillomania (Hair-Pulling Disorder)
- **Skin Picking:** Excoriation (Skin-Picking) Disorder

Trauma and Stressor-Related Disorders Diagnostic Flowchart

Step 1: Exposure to a Traumatic Event?

- **Yes:** Go to Step 2.
- **No:** Consider other disorders.

Step 2: Duration of Symptoms?

- **Less than 1 month:** Acute Stress Disorder
- **More than 1 month:** Posttraumatic Stress Disorder (PTSD)

Step 3: Presence of Emotional or Behavioral Symptoms in Response to a Stressor?

- **Yes:** Go to Step 4.
- **No:** Consider other diagnoses.

Step 4: Symptoms Occur Within 3 Months of Stressor?

- **Yes:** Adjustment Disorders
- **No:** Re-evaluate for PTSD or Acute Stress Disorder

Psychotic Disorders Diagnostic Flowchart

Step 1: Presence of Delusions, Hallucinations, or Disorganized Speech?

- **Yes:** Go to Step 2.
- **No:** Consider other disorders.

Step 2: Duration of Symptoms?

- **Less than 1 month:** Brief Psychotic Disorder
- **1-6 months:** Schizophreniform Disorder
- **More than 6 months:** Schizophrenia

Step 3: Presence of Major Mood Episode?

- **Yes:** Schizoaffective Disorder
- **No:** Confirm Schizophrenia or Brief Psychotic Disorder based on duration.

Step 4: Presence of Only Delusions?

- **Yes:** Delusional Disorder
- **No:** Re-evaluate for Schizophrenia or other psychotic disorders.

Feeding and Eating Disorders Diagnostic Flowchart

Step 1: Significant Weight Loss or Distorted Body Image?

- **Yes:** Go to Step 2.
- **No:** Consider other disorders.

Step 2: Restriction of Energy Intake Relative to Requirements?

- **Yes:** Anorexia Nervosa
- **No:** Go to Step 3.

Step 3: Recurrent Episodes of Binge Eating?

- **Yes:** Go to Step 4.
- **No:** Consider Avoidant/Restrictive Food Intake Disorder (ARFID)

Step 4: Compensatory Behaviors to Prevent Weight Gain?

- **Yes:** Bulimia Nervosa
- **No:** Binge-Eating Disorder

Dissociative Disorders Diagnostic Flowchart

Step 1: Presence of Dissociative Symptoms?

- **Yes:** Go to Step 2.
- **No:** Consider other disorders.

Step 2: Sudden Inability to Recall Important Personal Information?

- **Yes:** Dissociative Amnesia
- **No:** Go to Step 3.

Step 3: Experience of Two or More Distinct Personality States?

- **Yes:** Dissociative Identity Disorder (DID)
- **No:** Depersonalization/Derealization Disorder

Somatic Symptom and Related Disorders Diagnostic Flowchart

Step 1: Presence of Somatic Symptoms?

- **Yes:** Go to Step 2.
- **No:** Consider other disorders.

Step 2: Excessive Thoughts, Feelings, or Behaviors Related to Somatic Symptoms?

- **Yes:** Somatic Symptom Disorder
- **No:** Consider subclinical somatic symptoms.

Step 3: Preoccupation with Having or Acquiring a Serious Illness?

- **Yes:** Illness Anxiety Disorder
- **No:** Consider Conversion Disorder

Step 4: Falsification of Symptoms without Obvious External Incentives?

- **Yes:** Factitious Disorder
- **No:** Re-evaluate for other somatic symptom-related disorders.

Sleep-Wake Disorders Diagnostic Flowchart

Step 1: Difficulty Initiating or Maintaining Sleep?

- **Yes:** Go to Step 2.
- **No:** Consider other sleep disorders.

Step 2: Daytime Fatigue or Sleepiness?

- **Yes:** Insomnia Disorder
- **No:** Go to Step 3.

Step 3: Excessive Daytime Sleepiness Despite Adequate Sleep?

- **Yes:** Hypersomnolence Disorder
- **No:** Go to Step 4.

Step 4: Recurrent Episodes of Irresistible Sleep?

- **Yes:** Narcolepsy
- **No:** Consider other sleep-wake disorders.

Step 5: Breathing-Related Sleep Issues?

- **Yes:** Evaluate for Sleep Apnea
- **No:** Go to Step 6.

Step 6: Disruption of Sleep Due to Circadian Rhythm Issues?

- **Yes:** Circadian Rhythm Sleep-Wake Disorder
- **No:** Consider Parasomnias

Sexual Dysfunctions Diagnostic Flowchart

Step 1: Difficulty in Sexual Response Cycle?

- **Yes:** Go to Step 2.
- **No:** Consider other disorders.

Step 2: Desire Phase Issues?

- **Yes:** Male Hypoactive Sexual Desire Disorder or Female Sexual Interest/Arousal Disorder
- **No:** Go to Step 3.

Step 3: Arousal Phase Issues?

- **Yes:** Erectile Disorder (in males) or Female Sexual Interest/Arousal Disorder
- **No:** Go to Step 4.

Step 4: Orgasm Phase Issues?

- **Yes:** Premature Ejaculation, Delayed Ejaculation, or Female Orgasmic Disorder
- **No:** Go to Step 5.

Step 5: Pain During Intercourse?

- **Yes:** Genito-Pelvic Pain/Penetration Disorder
- **No:** Re-evaluate symptoms and consider differential diagnoses.

Disruptive, Impulse-Control, and Conduct Disorders Diagnostic Flowchart

Step 1: Persistent Pattern of Angry/Irritable Mood, Argumentative/Defiant Behavior, or Vindictiveness?

- **Yes:** Oppositional Defiant Disorder (ODD)
- **No:** Go to Step 2.

Step 2: Recurrent Outbursts Representing a Failure to Control Aggressive Impulses?

- **Yes:** Intermittent Explosive Disorder
- **No:** Go to Step 3.

Step 3: Persistent Pattern of Behavior that Violates the Basic Rights of Others or Major Age-Appropriate Societal Norms?

- **Yes:** Conduct Disorder
- **No:** Re-evaluate for other disruptive, impulse-control, and conduct disorders.

Substance-Related and Addictive Disorders Diagnostic Flowchart

Step 1: Use of Substance?

- **Yes:** Go to Step 2.
- **No:** Consider other disorders.

Step 2: Pattern of Substance Use Leading to Significant Impairment or Distress?

- **Yes:** Substance Use Disorder
- **No:** Consider other substance-related disorders.

Step 3: Presence of Tolerance or Withdrawal Symptoms?

- **Yes:** Substance Dependence
- **No:** Go to Step 4.

Step 4: Persistent Desire or Unsuccessful Efforts to Cut Down or Control Substance Use?

- **Yes:** Substance Use Disorder

- **No:** Consider Substance Intoxication or Substance Withdrawal

Step 5: Behavioral Symptoms Related to Gambling?

- **Yes:** Gambling Disorder
- **No:** Re-evaluate for Substance Use Disorder

Neurocognitive Disorders Diagnostic Flowchart

Step 1: Evidence of Cognitive Decline from a Previous Level of Performance?

- **Yes:** Go to Step 2.
- **No:** Consider other disorders.

Step 2: Interference with Independence in Everyday Activities?

- **Yes:** Major Neurocognitive Disorder
- **No:** Mild Neurocognitive Disorder

Step 3: Rule Out Delirium?

- **Yes:** Proceed with diagnosis
- **No:** Diagnose Delirium if criteria met

Step 4: Determine Etiology (e.g., Alzheimer's, Vascular, Lewy Bodies)?

- **Yes:** Specify Etiology
- **No:** Conduct further assessment to determine etiology

Personality Disorders Diagnostic Flowchart

Step 1: Pattern of Inner Experience and Behavior Deviating Markedly from the Expectations of the Individual's Culture?

- **Yes:** Go to Step 2.
- **No:** Consider other disorders.

Step 2: Pervasive and Inflexible Patterns?

- **Yes:** Go to Step 3.
- **No:** Consider situational or temporary conditions.

Step 3: Onset in Adolescence or Early Adulthood?

- **Yes:** Go to Step 4.
- **No:** Consider other developmental or psychiatric conditions.

Step 4: Significant Distress or Impairment?

- **Yes:** Personality Disorder
- **No:** Consider subclinical traits or other disorders.

Step 5: Determine Specific Type (e.g., Borderline, Antisocial, Narcissistic)?

- **Yes:** Specify Type
- **No:** Re-evaluate symptoms and consider differential diagnoses.

Neurodevelopmental Disorders Diagnostic Flowchart

Step 1: Developmental Deficits Present?

- **Yes:** Go to Step 2.
- **No:** Consider other disorders.

Step 2: Communication Deficits or Social Interaction Impairments?

- **Yes:** Autism Spectrum Disorder (ASD) or Social (Pragmatic) Communication Disorder
- **No:** Go to Step 3.

Step 3: Motor Skills or Coordination Issues?

- **Yes:** Developmental Coordination Disorder or Stereotypic Movement Disorder
- **No:** Go to Step 4.

Step 4: Specific Learning Difficulties?

- **Yes:** Specific Learning Disorder
- **No:** Consider Intellectual Disability or Global Developmental Delay

Step 5: Attention Deficit and Hyperactivity Symptoms?

- **Yes:** Attention-Deficit/Hyperactivity Disorder (ADHD)
- **No:** Re-evaluate symptoms and consider differential diagnoses.

Disruptive, Impulse-Control, and Conduct Disorders Diagnostic Flowchart

Step 1: Persistent Pattern of Angry/Irritable Mood, Argumentative/Defiant Behavior, or Vindictiveness?

- **Yes:** Oppositional Defiant Disorder (ODD)
- **No:** Go to Step 2.

Step 2: Recurrent Outbursts Representing a Failure to Control Aggressive Impulses?

- **Yes:** Intermittent Explosive Disorder
- **No:** Go to Step 3.

Step 3: Persistent Pattern of Behavior that Violates the Basic Rights of Others or Major Age-Appropriate Societal Norms?

- **Yes:** Conduct Disorder
- **No:** Re-evaluate for other disruptive, impulse-control, and conduct disorders.

How to Create Diagnostic Flowcharts

Creating diagnostic flowcharts is an effective way to simplify and visualize the diagnostic process for various mental health disorders. These flowcharts can help clinicians, students, and other mental health professionals systematically assess symptoms and make accurate diagnoses based on DSM-5-TR criteria. Here's a step-by-step guide to creating diagnostic flowcharts:

Step-by-Step Guide to Creating Diagnostic Flowcharts

Step 1: Identify the Disorder Category

- Start by selecting the broad category of disorders you want to create a flowchart for, such as mood disorders, anxiety disorders, or neurodevelopmental disorders.

Step 2: Gather Diagnostic Criteria

- Review the DSM-5-TR criteria for the specific disorders within your chosen category. Pay attention to key symptoms, duration, and exclusion criteria.

Step 3: Outline Key Decision Points

- Identify the critical decision points that guide the diagnostic process. These typically include the presence of specific symptoms, the duration of symptoms, and the exclusion of other disorders.

221

Step 4: Arrange Decision Points Sequentially

- Arrange the decision points in a logical sequence, starting with the most general symptoms and progressing to more specific criteria. Ensure each step logically leads to the next.

Step 5: Create Visual Representation

- Use a flowchart tool or diagram software (such as Microsoft Visio, Lucidchart, or even PowerPoint) to visually map out the decision points. Use standard flowchart symbols such as rectangles for steps, diamonds for decision points, and arrows to indicate the flow.

Step 6: Add Labels and Explanations

- Clearly label each step and decision point. Add brief explanations or criteria to ensure clarity. For example, label a decision diamond with "Presence of Excessive Worry?" and provide criteria like "More than 6 months: GAD".

Step 7: Test and Refine

- Test the flowchart by applying it to real or hypothetical case scenarios. Make sure it accurately guides the user through the diagnostic process. Refine the flowchart based on feedback and practical use.

Sample Questions

Here are 30 practice questions based on the DSM-5-TR criteria, covering various disorders. These questions are designed to test your understanding of diagnostic criteria, treatment options, and key features of different mental health conditions.

Practice Questions

1. **Major Depressive Disorder** A 35-year-old woman reports feeling extremely sad for the past month, losing interest in activities she used to enjoy, and experiencing significant weight loss. She also mentions having trouble sleeping and concentrating at work. Which of the following is the most likely diagnosis?

   A) Generalized Anxiety Disorder

   B) Major Depressive Disorder

   C) Bipolar I Disorder

   D) Persistent Depressive Disorder

2. **Generalized Anxiety Disorder** A 28-year-old man presents with excessive worry about various aspects of his life, including work and relationships. He finds it difficult to control his worry, experiences muscle tension, and has trouble sleeping.

These symptoms have been present for the past eight months. What is the most appropriate diagnosis?

A) Panic Disorder

B) Social Anxiety Disorder

C) Generalized Anxiety Disorder

D) Obsessive-Compulsive Disorder

3. **Schizophrenia** A 22-year-old man reports hearing voices that comment on his actions, having delusions that people are spying on him, and exhibiting disorganized speech. These symptoms have been present for the past seven months. What is the most likely diagnosis?

A) Brief Psychotic Disorder

B) Schizoaffective Disorder

C) Schizophrenia

D) Delusional Disorder

4. **Posttraumatic Stress Disorder** A 30-year-old woman who survived a severe car accident six months ago reports having frequent nightmares about the accident, avoiding driving, and feeling constantly on edge. What is the most appropriate diagnosis?

A) Acute Stress Disorder

B) Adjustment Disorder

C) Generalized Anxiety Disorder

D) Posttraumatic Stress Disorder

5. **Obsessive-Compulsive Disorder** A 25-year-old woman reports that she spends hours each day washing her hands and cleaning her house to get rid of "contaminants." She recognizes that her fears are excessive but feels unable to stop. Which of the following is the most likely diagnosis?

A) Specific Phobia

B) Generalized Anxiety Disorder

C) Obsessive-Compulsive Disorder

D) Illness Anxiety Disorder

6. **Bipolar I Disorder** A 40-year-old man experiences episodes of elevated mood, increased energy, and decreased need for sleep that last for about a week, followed by periods of deep depression. What is the most appropriate diagnosis?

A) Major Depressive Disorder

B) Bipolar I Disorder

C) Cyclothymic Disorder

D) Persistent Depressive Disorder

7. **Social Anxiety Disorder** A 21-year-old college student avoids giving presentations in class and declines social invitations due to intense fear of being judged or embarrassed. This fear has been present for over a year and causes significant distress. What is the most likely diagnosis?

A) Panic Disorder

B) Generalized Anxiety Disorder

C) Social Anxiety Disorder

D) Specific Phobia

8. **Panic Disorder** A 32-year-old woman experiences sudden episodes of intense fear, heart palpitations, sweating, trembling, and a fear of losing control. These episodes occur unexpectedly and have been happening for the past six months. What is the most appropriate diagnosis?

A) Specific Phobia

B) Generalized Anxiety Disorder

C) Panic Disorder

D) Social Anxiety Disorder

9. **Specific Phobia** A 29-year-old man avoids flying due to an intense fear of airplane crashes. The fear is so severe that it interferes with his ability to travel for work. Which of the following is the most likely diagnosis?

A) Generalized Anxiety Disorder

B) Panic Disorder

C) Agoraphobia

D) Specific Phobia

10. **Attention-Deficit/Hyperactivity Disorder (ADHD)** A 10-year-old boy has difficulty paying attention in class, often fidgets, interrupts others, and has trouble completing assignments. These behaviors have been present for over six months and are causing problems at school and home. What is the most likely diagnosis?

A) Oppositional Defiant Disorder

B) Generalized Anxiety Disorder

C) Attention-Deficit/Hyperactivity Disorder

D) Specific Learning Disorder

11. **Anorexia Nervosa** A 17-year-old girl has significantly reduced her food intake, leading to a dangerously low body weight. She expresses an intense fear of gaining

weight and a distorted body image. What is the most appropriate diagnosis?

A) Bulimia Nervosa

B) Binge-Eating Disorder

C) Anorexia Nervosa

D) Avoidant/Restrictive Food Intake Disorder

12. **Bulimia Nervosa** A 19-year-old woman reports episodes of binge eating followed by self-induced vomiting to prevent weight gain. These episodes occur at least twice a week for the past three months. What is the most likely diagnosis?

A) Anorexia Nervosa

B) Binge-Eating Disorder

C) Avoidant/Restrictive Food Intake Disorder

D) Bulimia Nervosa

13. **Binge-Eating Disorder** A 24-year-old man experiences recurrent episodes of eating large amounts of food in a short period, during which he feels a lack of control. He does not engage in compensatory behaviors like purging. What is the most appropriate diagnosis?

A) Bulimia Nervosa

B) Anorexia Nervosa

C) Binge-Eating Disorder

D) Avoidant/Restrictive Food Intake Disorder

14. **Oppositional Defiant Disorder (ODD)** A 9-year-old boy frequently argues with adults, refuses to comply with rules, and deliberately annoys others. These behaviors have been present for at least six months. What is the most likely diagnosis?

A) Conduct Disorder

B) Attention-Deficit/Hyperactivity Disorder

C) Oppositional Defiant Disorder

D) Intermittent Explosive Disorder

15. **Conduct Disorder** A 16-year-old boy has a history of aggressive behavior towards people and animals, destruction of property, deceitfulness, and serious rule violations. These behaviors have been present for over a year. What is the most appropriate diagnosis?

A) Oppositional Defiant Disorder

B) Attention-Deficit/Hyperactivity Disorder

C) Conduct Disorder

D) Intermittent Explosive Disorder

16. **Borderline Personality Disorder (BPD)** A 25-year-old woman exhibits unstable relationships, impulsive behaviors, intense fear of abandonment, and recurrent self-harming actions. These symptoms have been present for several years. What is the most likely diagnosis?

A) Histrionic Personality Disorder

B) Borderline Personality Disorder

C) Narcissistic Personality Disorder

D) Avoidant Personality Disorder

17. **Antisocial Personality Disorder** A 30-year-old man has a history of disregard for the rights of others, deceitfulness, impulsivity, irritability, and lack of remorse for his actions. These behaviors began in adolescence. What is the most appropriate diagnosis?

A) Borderline Personality Disorder

B) Narcissistic Personality Disorder

C) Histrionic Personality Disorder

D) Antisocial Personality Disorder

18. **Narcissistic Personality Disorder** A 35-year-old man exhibits grandiosity, a need for excessive admiration, and a lack of empathy for others. He has a sense of entitlement and is often envious of others. What is the most likely diagnosis?

A) Borderline Personality Disorder

B) Narcissistic Personality Disorder

C) Histrionic Personality Disorder

D) Antisocial Personality Disorder

19. **Histrionic Personality Disorder** A 28-year-old woman is characterized by excessive emotionality, attention-seeking behavior, and a need to be the center of attention. She often uses her physical appearance to draw attention to herself. What is the most appropriate diagnosis?

A) Borderline Personality Disorder

B) Narcissistic Personality Disorder

C) Histrionic Personality Disorder

D) Antisocial Personality Disorder

20. **Avoidant Personality Disorder** A 32-year-old man avoids social interactions due to fears of criticism, disapproval, or rejection. He perceives himself as socially inept and inferior to others. What is the most likely diagnosis?

A) Schizoid Personality Disorder

B) Avoidant Personality Disorder

C) Dependent Personality Disorder

D) Obsessive-Compulsive Personality Disorder

21. **Dependent Personality Disorder** A 40-year-old woman has an excessive need to be taken care of, leading to submissive and clinging behaviors. She has difficulty making decisions without reassurance from others and fears being left to take care of herself. What is the most appropriate diagnosis?

A) Borderline Personality Disorder

B) Avoidant Personality Disorder

C) Dependent Personality Disorder

D) Histrionic Personality Disorder

22. **Obsessive-Compulsive Personality Disorder** A 45-year-old man is preoccupied with orderliness, perfectionism, and control. He often becomes so focused

on details that he cannot complete tasks. He finds it difficult to delegate tasks to others. What is the most likely diagnosis?

A) Obsessive-Compulsive Disorder

B) Narcissistic Personality Disorder

C) Obsessive-Compulsive Personality Disorder

D) Borderline Personality Disorder

23. **Schizoid Personality Disorder** A 38-year-old woman has a long history of social detachment and prefers solitary activities. She shows little interest in forming personal relationships and appears emotionally cold. What is the most likely diagnosis?

A) Avoidant Personality Disorder

B) Schizoid Personality Disorder

C) Schizotypal Personality Disorder

D) Borderline Personality Disorder

24. **Schizotypal Personality Disorder** A 29-year-old man exhibits odd beliefs, unusual perceptual experiences, and eccentric behavior. He has few close friends and displays inappropriate or constricted affect. What is the most appropriate diagnosis?

A) Schizoid Personality Disorder

B) Schizotypal Personality Disorder

C) Avoidant Personality Disorder

D) Borderline Personality Disorder

25. **Delusional Disorder** A 45-year-old woman believes that she is being followed by a secret organization that wants to harm her. She holds this belief despite lack of evidence and has been experiencing these delusions for the past six months. What is the most likely diagnosis?

A) Schizophrenia

B) Brief Psychotic Disorder

C) Delusional Disorder

D) Schizoaffective Disorder

26. **Brief Psychotic Disorder** A 22-year-old woman experiences hallucinations and disorganized speech following a stressful event. These symptoms last for three weeks and then completely resolve. What is the most appropriate diagnosis?

A) Schizophrenia

B) Brief Psychotic Disorder

C) Schizoaffective Disorder

D) Delusional Disorder

27. **Schizoaffective Disorder** A 30-year-old man has a combination of symptoms from schizophrenia, such as hallucinations, and mood disorder symptoms, like depression, that occur simultaneously. What is the most likely diagnosis?

A) Schizophrenia

B) Bipolar Disorder

C) Schizoaffective Disorder

D) Delusional Disorder

28. **Cyclothymic Disorder** A 35-year-old woman experiences numerous periods of hypomanic symptoms and periods of depressive symptoms that do not meet the criteria for major depressive episodes. These symptoms have persisted for over two years. What is the most appropriate diagnosis?

A) Bipolar I Disorder

B) Bipolar II Disorder

C) Cyclothymic Disorder

D) Major Depressive Disorder

29. **Persistent Depressive Disorder (Dysthymia)** A 40-year-old man has felt consistently low in mood for the past three years. Although his symptoms are less severe than major depression, they are persistent and affect his daily functioning. What is the most likely diagnosis?

A) Major Depressive Disorder

B) Persistent Depressive Disorder

C) Bipolar II Disorder

D) Cyclothymic Disorder

30. **Illness Anxiety Disorder** A 28-year-old woman frequently visits her doctor, fearing she has serious illnesses despite having no significant medical findings. Her preoccupation with health causes significant distress and impairment. What is the most likely diagnosis?

A) Somatic Symptom Disorder

B) Illness Anxiety Disorder

C) Factitious Disorder

D) Conversion Disorder

Answer Key and Explanations

1. **Answer:** B) Major Depressive Disorder

   Explanation: The patient's symptoms of persistent sadness, loss of interest in activities, significant weight loss, insomnia, and concentration difficulties for over two weeks are characteristic of Major Depressive Disorder (MDD).

2. **Answer:** C) Generalized Anxiety Disorder

   Explanation: The patient's excessive worry about multiple areas of his life, difficulty controlling the worry, muscle tension, and sleep disturbances for more than six months are indicative of Generalized Anxiety Disorder (GAD).

3. **Answer:** C) Schizophrenia

   Explanation: The patient's auditory hallucinations, delusions, and disorganized speech for more than six months fit the criteria for Schizophrenia.

4. **Answer:** D) Posttraumatic Stress Disorder

   Explanation: The patient's symptoms of re-experiencing the traumatic event (nightmares), avoidance behavior, and hyperarousal (feeling on edge) for more than one month suggest Posttraumatic Stress Disorder (PTSD).

5. **Answer:** C) Obsessive-Compulsive Disorder

   Explanation: The patient's excessive hand washing and cleaning, along with recognition of her fears as excessive but feeling unable to stop, indicate Obsessive-Compulsive Disorder (OCD).

6. **Answer:** B) Bipolar I Disorder

   Explanation: The patient's episodes of elevated mood, increased energy, decreased need for sleep, and periods of depression fit the criteria for Bipolar I Disorder.

7. **Answer:** C) Social Anxiety Disorder

Explanation: The patient's intense fear of social judgment, avoidance of social situations, and significant distress for over a year are characteristic of Social Anxiety Disorder.

8. **Answer:** C) Panic Disorder

Explanation: The patient's sudden episodes of intense fear, heart palpitations, sweating, and fear of losing control for six months are indicative of Panic Disorder.

9. **Answer:** D) Specific Phobia

Explanation: The patient's intense fear of flying, avoidance behavior, and significant impairment in functioning fit the criteria for Specific Phobia.

10. **Answer:** C) Attention-Deficit/Hyperactivity Disorder

Explanation: The boy's difficulty paying attention, fidgeting, interrupting others, and trouble completing assignments for over six months are indicative of ADHD.

11. **Answer:** C) Anorexia Nervosa

Explanation: The patient's significant weight loss, intense fear of gaining weight, and distorted body image indicate Anorexia Nervosa.

12. **Answer:** D) Bulimia Nervosa

Explanation: The patient's recurrent episodes of binge eating followed by compensatory behaviors (vomiting) for at least three months fit the criteria for Bulimia Nervosa.

13. **Answer:** C) Binge-Eating Disorder

Explanation: The patient's recurrent episodes of binge eating without compensatory behaviors, and associated distress, indicate Binge-Eating Disorder.

14. **Answer:** C) Oppositional Defiant Disorder

Explanation: The boy's frequent arguments with adults, refusal to comply with rules, and deliberate annoyance of others for at least six months suggest Oppositional Defiant Disorder.

15. **Answer:** C) Conduct Disorder

Explanation: The boy's aggressive behavior, destruction of property, deceitfulness, and serious rule violations for over a year are indicative of Conduct Disorder.

16. **Answer:** B) Borderline Personality Disorder

Explanation: The patient's unstable relationships, impulsive behaviors, fear of abandonment, and recurrent self-harm indicate Borderline Personality Disorder.

17. **Answer:** D) Antisocial Personality Disorder

Explanation: The patient's history of disregard for others' rights, deceitfulness, impulsivity, irritability, and lack of remorse beginning in adolescence fit the criteria for Antisocial Personality Disorder.

18. **Answer:** B) Narcissistic Personality Disorder

Explanation: The patient's grandiosity, need for excessive admiration, lack of empathy, and sense of entitlement indicate Narcissistic Personality Disorder.

19. **Answer:** C) Histrionic Personality Disorder

Explanation: The patient's excessive emotionality, attention-seeking behavior, and need to be the center of attention fit the criteria for Histrionic Personality Disorder.

20. **Answer:** B) Avoidant Personality Disorder

Explanation: The patient's avoidance of social interactions due to fears of criticism and rejection, and feelings of social ineptness indicate Avoidant Personality Disorder.

21. **Answer:** C) Dependent Personality Disorder

Explanation: The patient's excessive need to be taken care of, submissive and clinging behaviors, and difficulty making decisions without reassurance fit the criteria for Dependent Personality Disorder.

22. **Answer:** C) Obsessive-Compulsive Personality Disorder

Explanation: The patient's preoccupation with orderliness, perfectionism, and control, and difficulty delegating tasks, indicate Obsessive-Compulsive Personality Disorder.

23. **Answer:** B) Schizoid Personality Disorder

Explanation: The patient's social detachment, preference for solitary activities, and emotional coldness fit the criteria for Schizoid Personality Disorder.

24. **Answer:** B) Schizotypal Personality Disorder

Explanation: The patient's odd beliefs, unusual perceptual experiences, eccentric behavior, and few close friends indicate Schizotypal Personality Disorder.

25. **Answer:** C) Delusional Disorder

Explanation: The patient's persistent delusions of being followed by a secret organization for six months without other psychotic symptoms fit the criteria for Delusional Disorder.

26. **Answer:** B) Brief Psychotic Disorder

Explanation: The patient's hallucinations and disorganized speech following a stressful event, lasting for three weeks and then resolving, indicate Brief Psychotic Disorder.

27. **Answer:** C) Schizoaffective Disorder

Explanation: The patient's combination of schizophrenia symptoms (hallucinations and delusions) along with mood disorder symptoms (depression or mania) that occur simultaneously suggest Schizoaffective Disorder.

28. **Answer:** C) Cyclothymic Disorder

Explanation: The patient's numerous periods of hypomanic symptoms and depressive symptoms that do not meet criteria for major depressive episodes, persisting for over two years, fit the criteria for Cyclothymic Disorder.

29. **Answer:** B) Persistent Depressive Disorder

Explanation: The patient's consistent low mood for the past three years, less severe than major depression but persistent and affecting daily functioning, indicates Persistent Depressive Disorder (Dysthymia).

30. **Answer:** B) Illness Anxiety Disorder

Explanation: The patient's frequent visits to the doctor due to fear of serious illnesses, despite no significant medical findings, and preoccupation with health causing significant distress, fit the criteria for Illness Anxiety Disorder.

PART IV:

Online and Interactive Resources

Overview

The online and interactive resources are designed to complement the study guide and provide additional tools to enhance your learning experience. These resources include quizzes, flashcards, and audio summaries that are accessible through the dedicated website for this study guide. Utilizing these resources will help reinforce your understanding of the DSM-5-TR material, making your study process more efficient and effective.

Components of Online and Interactive Resources

1. **Quizzes**
2. **Flashcards**
3. **Audio Summaries**

1. Quizzes

Description:
- Interactive quizzes for each chapter and major disorder category.
- Designed to test your knowledge and understanding of the DSM-5-TR criteria and concepts.
- Immediate feedback with explanations for each answer to help you learn from your mistakes.

Access:

- Quizzes are available online and can be accessed through the study guide's website.
- Organized by chapter and disorder category to allow targeted practice.

QR Code Access:

- Scan the QR code below to access the quizzes:

2. Flashcards

Description:

- Interactive flashcards for quick review and memorization.
- Each flashcard includes key symptoms, diagnostic criteria, and treatment options for major DSM-5-TR disorders.
- Useful for on-the-go study and quick revision sessions.

Access:

- Flashcards can be accessed online through the study guide's website.
- Digital versions are optimized for use on computers, tablets, and smartphones.

QR Code Access:

- Scan the QR code below to access the flashcards:

3. Audio Summaries

Description:

- Audio summaries for each chapter and major disorder category.
- Provides an overview of key concepts, diagnostic criteria, and treatment options.
- Ideal for auditory learners and for reinforcing material during commutes or downtime.

Access:

- Audio summaries are available for streaming through the study guide's website.
- Organized by chapter and disorder category for easy navigation.

QR Code Access:

- Scan the QR code below to access the audio summaries:

PART V:

Conclusion and Additional Resources

Conclusion

The journey through the DSM-5-TR is both challenging and rewarding. This study guide aims to simplify complex diagnostic criteria, enhance understanding through mnemonics and flowcharts, and provide comprehensive practice through quizzes and case studies. As you continue to delve into the nuances of mental health diagnosis and treatment, remember the importance of continuous learning and staying updated with the latest research and clinical practices.

Additional Resources

To further support your learning and professional development, we recommend the following additional resources:

1. **Books and Textbooks**
   - *DSM-5-TR® Self-Exam Questions* by Maalobeeka Gangopadhyay, Philip R. Muskin, Anna L. Dickerman, Andrew Drysdale, Claire C. Holderness. This book provides extensive practice questions and detailed explanations.
   - *Kaplan & Sadock's Synopsis of Psychiatry* by Benjamin J. Sadock, Virginia A. Sadock, and Pedro Ruiz. A comprehensive resource for psychiatric conditions, treatment, and research.

2. **Online Courses and Webinars**
   - **Coursera**: Offers courses on psychological disorders, therapeutic approaches, and clinical psychology from leading universities.
   - **Udemy**: Provides affordable courses on DSM-5-TR, mental health diagnostics, and psychotherapy techniques.

3. **Professional Organizations**
   - **American Psychiatric Association (APA)**: Offers resources, continuing education, and professional guidelines for psychiatrists and mental health professionals.
   - **National Alliance on Mental Illness (NAMI)**: Provides educational resources, support networks, and advocacy for individuals affected by mental illness.

4. **Journals and Research Databases**
   - **PubMed**: A free database of biomedical and life sciences literature, providing access to research articles and clinical studies.
   - **PsychiatryOnline**: Offers access to journals, books, and practice guidelines published by the American Psychiatric Association.

5. **Mobile Apps**
   - **Medscape**: Provides access to medical news, clinical references, and professional education.
   - **PsycEssentials**: A handy reference tool for DSM-5 criteria and diagnostic information.

QR Codes for Online Resources

Access our comprehensive online resources through the QR codes provided below:

Quizzes:

- Scan the QR code to access interactive quizzes designed to test your knowledge and understanding of DSM-5-TR criteria and concepts.

Flashcards:

- Scan the QR code to access interactive flashcards for quick review and memorization of key symptoms, diagnostic criteria, and treatment options.

Audio Summaries:

- Scan the QR code to access audio summaries that provide overviews of key concepts, diagnostic criteria, and treatment options for auditory learners.

Made in the USA
Las Vegas, NV
13 December 2024

14008341R00144